# The Heart
# Transmission
# of Medicine

# The Heart Transmission of Medicine

by Liu Yi-ren

translated by
Yang Shou-zhong

BLUE POPPY PRESS

Published by:

**BLUE POPPY PRESS, INC.**
**1775 LINDEN AVE.**
**BOULDER, CO 80304**

**First Edition, June, 1997**

ISBN 0-936185-83-X
LC 97-70142

The information in this book is given in good faith. However, the
translators and the publishers cannot be held responsible for any error or
omission. Nor can they be held in any way responsible for treatment given
on the basis of information contained in this book. The publishers make
this information available to English language readers for scholarly and
research purposes only.

The publishers do not advocate nor endorse self-medication by laypersons.
Chinese medicine is a professional medicine. Laypersons interested in
availing themselves of the treatments described in this book should seek
out a qualified professional practitioner of Chinese medicine.

COMP Designation: Denotative translation

Printed at Johnson Printing in Boulder, CO
on essentially chlorine-free paper
Cover calligraphy by Michael Sullivan (Seiho)
Cover design by Bob Schram, Bookends Design

10 9 8 7 6 5 4 3 2 1

# Translator's Foreword

This book was written by Liu Yi-ren. We know literally nothing about the author except that he lived during the reign of Dao Guang (1821-1851 CE), the sixth emperor of the Qing dynasty. This book is a condensed primer on Chinese medicine and particularly on treating the most common traditional Chinese disease categories with Chinese medicinals. As such, it is an excellent abridged guide for students and a handy reference for clinicians.

To become a doctor in old China, one had to apprentice for many years under the personal guidance of a mentor-physician. During the first years of apprenticeship, all one's days were spent running errands and doing all sorts of chores seemingly irrevelant to the practice of medicine. If one's performance as an obedient servant proved satisfactory, then one might be allowed to begin studying medicine *per se*. This second period of training was no less arduous than the first. At first, one simply had to sit by the side of the master while he received his patients, watching and listening to the master and copying his prescriptions. In his spare time, the student was required to memorize oceans of formulas and the subtle differences of signs and symptoms of innumerable diseases. Such traditional apprenticeships typically lasted more than 10 years. Only after that was the student allowed to start seeing patients by themselves.

After Liberation (*i.e.*, 1949), this traditional medical educational system was completely transformed. The above-described one-on-one method of instruction was largely abandoned. Special schools of Chinese medicine have been set up throughout China which can accommodate hundreds or even thousands of times more students than in the past. This has made it possible to not only mass produce qualified physicians but also to introduce modern concepts and methods of education. Medical students are no longer required to do their teachers' household chores and everyday tasks. However, the laborious task of learning all of the sophisticated theories of Chinese medicine and a repertoire of medicinal formulas still remains.

Therefore, in the present as in the past, students of Chinese medicine still need a single book which contains the most complicated theories in easy words and short passages. Unlike the classics which may be a challenge even to learned scholars, what has perennially been wanted is a book which is accessible to beginners who have only a rudimentary knowledge of traditional Chinese medicine. In addition, it would be a blessing for students of Chinese medicine if one only had to memorize a handful of formulas rather than myriads.

In response to this ongoing need, many contemporary as well as past scholars have attempted to compile easy readers of Chinese medicine to reduce the difficulty of learning this complex art. However, rarely have the authors of such primers escaped the blame of erroneously oversimplifying the coherent, grand system of traditional Chinese medicine. The crux of the issue has always been to create a concise work without throwing the baby out with the bathwater. On the other hand, some premodern works, like the *Yi Xue Ru Men (Entering the Gate of Medicine)*, which, judging from their titles, seem like primers for beginners, are, in fact, too volumious for beginning students' needs.

Therefore, few of these efforts are truly recommendable. This present work is one of the few successes within this genre. First of all, this work is a primer in its true sense. It is not a difficult job to memorize such a thin book by heart. More importantly, this book contains the very essence of Chinese medicine. Since the material in this book is undiluted, it can come in a small package.

Take the introduction of formulas for example. The *Zhong Yi Da Ci Dian (A Dictionary of Chinese Medicine)*'s volume on formulas and prescriptions ("*Fang Ji Fen Ce*"), published by the People's Public Health Press in 1983. It contains 7,500 medicinal formulas. This is a prodigious number. It is lucky that practitioners of Chinese medicine need not memorize all these thousands of formulas. It is said that the number in common clinical use is about 300. But even just these 300 or so formulas take a lot of time and energy to learn.

However, the author of this current work picks only a handful of the most famous formulas as the signposts for the basis of formulary design. One can then derive a series of related formulas from each of these few basic formulas by making all sorts of additions and subtractions. Equipped with the fundamental theoretical knowledge of Chinese medicine which Liu presents in a condensed yet systematic way, one is able to modify a limited number of formulas to successfully cope with the multifarious diseases encountered in clinical practice. This practice of the author reminds us of the great physician, Zhu Zhen-heng (a.k.a. Zhu Dan-xi, 1281-1358 CE), who also sytematized medical formulas in a similar way.[1]

Because of this book's strong points noted above, it immediately became popular among Chinese physicians and their students. This is evidenced by the fact that it has been published time and time again. In addition, this book is still used in New China today. In some provinces, it is a required text for students and junior physicians. No other premodern medical work, however great, has secured such a prestigious position in the field of entry level education. Initially, this book was published in New China under the name *Zhong Yi Jie Jing (A Short Cut to Chinese Medicine)*. The substitution of this title underscores how suitable teachers of Chinese medicine in China have found this book to be for beginners.

A part of this work, mainly that part dealing with the composition of formulas, was written in verse in order to make it easier for students to memorize. Unfortunately, we have not been able to preserve this style when translating this work into English. Honestly speaking, these verses are not, from a literary point of view, that well worded. In most cases, the only difference between these "verses" and how they would be written as prose is that they use only single ideograms as abbreviations of bi-or

---

[1]   Interested readers may compare Liu's approach to Zhu's in his *Dan Xi Xin Fa Zhi Yao (The Heart & Essence of Dan-xi's Methods of Treatment)*, Blue Poppy Press, Boulder, CO, 1993.

tri-character words. In other words, we have changed nothing in the translation except for the choice of the commonly used words in place of their abbreviations.

This translation is based on the version published by the Hebei People's Press in 1977. Those parts in square brackets are insertions made by the editors of the Chinese version rather than the translator unless those brackets are found within normal parentheses. The terminology in this translation is based on Nigel Wiseman's *English-Chinese, Chinese-English Dictionary of Chinese Medicine* published by the Hunan Science & Technology Press, Changsha, 1995. Formulas are identified by their Pinyin names followed by their English translation. Medicinal identifications are based on Bensky & Gamble's *Herbal Medicine: Materia Medica* and the Shanghai Science & Technology Press's *Zhong Yao Da Ci Dian (Encyclopedia of Chinese Medicinals)*. This means that the translator consulted the first title first. If the medicinal in question was not found in that book, the translator then consulted the second book.

Yang Shou-zhong
North China Coal Mines Medical College
Tangshan, Hebei

# Foreword[1]

1. One should first become familiar with the first 13 chapters of the hand-copied *Heart Transmission*.[2]

After one has read the chapter, "Prose & Verse Transmitting the Heart of Using Medicinals" (Ch. 7), one should have a rough idea about the natures of medicinals. After one has read the chapter, "Rhymes on the Ruling Medicinals (Used) in Treating Disease" (Ch. 8), one will be equipped with a knowledge of the ruling medicinals for each of the various diseases. In "Channel Conducting Medicinals" (Ch. 6) there are (only) a couple of lines. (Each of) the hundreds of diseases involves a channel and network vessel and requires multitudes of medicinals. Without appropriate channel conductors, the many (other) medicinals (in a formula) can find nowhere to gather (after being taken into the body) and, hence, may contrarily do harm. This is like many people paying a visit without an usher. No one can find their way to the hall. (The same) is meant by the saying that a thread can do nothing without a needle.

After one has read the "Heart-imparting Rhymes on Pulse Examination" (Ch. 1), one will have a knowledge of the names and images of the pulses by which one can know the lightness or seriousness, the urgency or moderateness, the vacuity or repletion, exterior or interior (condition of diseases). After one has read the essay, "General Essentials of Pulse Examination" (Ch. 2), one will be able to recognize the pattern of a disease by feeling the pulse. After one has read the essay, "The Six Methods of Pulse Examination "(Ch. 3), one will be able to determine what types of pulse indicate no disease as regards the various parts (of the body). If the pulses are not such, one will know what kinds of disease there are in the

---

[1]  This foreword may have been written by the keeper of the work, Qian Le-tian, whose life story is also unknown.

[2]  Apparently, the original version of this work was circulated in hand-copied form.

various parts. After one has read the "Poem on the Study of the Three Positions as a Whole" (Ch. 4), one will know what the disease pattern is if one sees the same pulse (quality) in all three positions (on both hands).

After one has read the essay, "The Necessity of Rational Inquiry" (Ch. 5), one will be in command of the method of inquiry concerning disease.

There are five chapters (Ch. 9-13) on essential instructions on prescription. They deal with five decoctions.[3] Suppose one already has a rudimentary notion of the pulse, is informed on disease manifestations, and is equipped with a fundamental knowledge of the natures of medicinals, but one does not know the well-established formulas designed by the ancients or how to make additions and subtractions in accordance with particular cases. This is as good as abandoning the carpenter's line maker while intending to make an even plane of a curved plank or (it is like) putting aside the steelyard to weigh by hand. This will unavoidably lead to mistakes. To use the well-established formulas designed by the ancients, it is first necessary to examine the pulse to arrive at a knowledge of which viscera and bowels and which channels and network vessels are involved in the disease. Then one should use medicinals that can enter those (involved) channels and network vessels. In each formula, there are invariably a ruling medicinal, adjunct medicinals, and coordinators to match (the preceding two). The flavors of medicinals having undergone processing will change in nature. It is also possible that the medicinals in a formula may clash, fear, or aid each other. Therefore, (the ancients) never used these medicinals imprudently. They must have contemplated profoundly and comprehensively before they designed a well-established formula. They (then) made some additions and subtractions demonstrating to later students (exemplary) norms. If one is not well familiar with the natures of medicinals and does not know how to make additions and subtractions (to well-established formulas), one will, after examining the pulse, be at a loss how to construct a prescription.

---

[3] Because the majority of medicinal formulas are prepared in the form of decoction, formulas, whether prepared in the form of pills, powder, or decoction, are often simply called decoctions. In other words, in some contexts, the word decoction in Chinese is equivalent to the word formula.

The chapter, "Prose & Verse on Disease Causes" (Ch. 14), is most beautiful. If a person is taken with a pathocondition, (even though) it has its manifestations externally, one may be at a loss about how it is caused and ignorant of which viscera and bowels, channels and network vessels are damaged. If one is familiar with this chapter and if, after a study of the pulse, one is asked how the disease is caused and which viscera and bowels, channels and network vessels should be held responsible, one will be able to explain (all) this on the spot. This does not merely concern treating others. When one feels ill, one (who is furnished with this knowledge) may know the cause and (thereby) escape from the harm a vulgar healer may do one.

From the "Heart-imparting Rhymes on Pulse Examination" to the "Prose & Verse on Disease Causes", there are but 13 chapters which only take a number of days with which to become familiar. From there down, there are 74 (sub)chapters, each of which has a sentence from the "Prose & Verse on Disease Causes" as its title. Each (of these) chapters consists of a discussion of the cause of a (particular) disease and its treatment. For fear that people will not be able to memorize the ingredients of the prescribed decoctions, the medicinals of (each) formula are boiled down to a four-line stanza to facilitate learning. It is best if one learns the decoctions by heart. If not, one can go over them from time to time and, in due course, will have them at the tips of one's fingers.

There are more than 300 medicinals (in common use). In this book, they are divided into four categories: cold, hot, warm, and balanced. (However,) only 146 medicinals are included. Although this is less than half that number (*i.e.*, half of 300), it provides a sufficient number to choose from for practical use. In some cases, the nature of a medicinal is not fully illustrated, but a general idea of it is provided.

The essential teachings of the ancients provide a grand outline to medicine, but they are kept as secrets, and books on them are not available in the market. (Therefore,) it will suffice to pore over (but) this one book. Then one will not commit blunders in diagnosing and treating people.

2. In addition, one should read the work, the *Tu Zhu Nan Jing Mai Jue (The Illustrated & Annotated Rhymes on the Pulse from the Classic of Difficulties)*[4], which consists of four thin books. The entire *dao* of medicine (depends) on the necessity of having a perfect knowledge of pulse theories, the viscera and bowels, channels and network vessels, and generating and restraining (relationships) between the five phases. This work specializes in the vessels and network vessels with illustrations and annotations. In it, the "Song of the Formulated Pulse Examination Methods", the "Song of the Five Viscera", the "Song of the Seven Exterior & Eight Interior [Pulses] in the Nine Positions", and "Song on How to Feel the Pulse with the Fingers" are all written in verse. It is best if one can learn them by heart. As to other parts, one is only expected to go over them time and again and, in due course, one may have them at the tips of one's fingers. In connection with the third book of this work, it contains detailed annotations in the *Nan Jing (The Classic of Difficulties)*. While reading it, one can place the first book by its side, simultaneously consulting it. This way one will become well informed.

3. Further, one should read Wang Ren-an's[5] *Ben Cao Bei Yao (The Essential Reference to Materia Medica)*. It consists of four or five books specifically discussing the natures of medicinals.(It comes) with a thin book, the *Tang Tou Ge Jue (Rhymes on Decoctions)* as an appendix. In this appendix, 300 or more formulas are included, divided into 20 categories. Each rhyme on a decoction consists of but several sentences. One should learn these by heart. In regard to the (countless) ancient formulas, it is impossible to explain each (and every one) of them. This book chooses only four to five formulas for (each) of the most intractable bad diseases from the *Shang Han ([The Treatise on] Cold Damage)* with a view to demonstrating how to

---

[4] The author of this work was Zhang Shi-xian who lived in the 16th century. However, the editor of the modern Chinese version from which this translation has been made may be mistaken in terms of this work. It may be two independent works rather than one single work. Zhang compiled two works. One was the *Mai Jing Tu Jie (The Illustrated & Annotated Classic of the Pulse)*. The other was the *Nan Jing Tu Jie (The Illustrated & Annotated Classic of Difficulties)*. However, both are generally regarded as poorly written works.

[5] Wang Ren-an, style name Wang Ang (1615-?), was an accomplished physician and prolific writer on medicine.

use medicinals. This way, (the presentation) is not complicated, and, hence, one can easily command (the prescription).

4. Yet further, one may read the *Yi Fang Ji Jie (The Collected Annotations on Medical Formulas)* compiled by Wang Ren-an. This work exclusively contains old formulas designed by the ancients. It illustrates how the ancients designed formulas in accordance with particular diseases, intimating the pith and essence of medicinal prescriptions. It gives a classification or identification of 22 categories (of formulas), supplementing and boosting, exterior effusing, ejection, internal attacking, exterior and interior (resolving), harmonizing, qi-rectifying, blood-rectifying, wind-dispelling, cold-dispelling, summerheat-clearing, dampness-disinhibiting, dryness-moistening, fire-draining, phlegm-eliminating, dispersing and abducting, contracting and astringing, worm-killing, eye-brightening, and (those for) welling abscess and sores, pregnancy and childbirth, and emergency aid. In terms of supplementing and boosting, etc, there are detailed annotations, and, for each formula, there are also detailed explanations. One does not have to learn these by heart, but one should go over them carefully several times.

The pulse may agree with the manifested symptoms. This is congruence between the pulse and the symptoms. (For such a condition,) it is easy to make out a prescription based on an (established) formula with certain additions and subtractions. If the pulse suggests one (category of disease) while the manifested symptoms imply another, this is disagreement between the pulse and the symptoms. A disease with such disagreement is usually difficult to treat. One should never prescribe medicinals presumptuously if, after examination, one is unable to diagnose the pattern of the affliction. Whether (based on) precedence of the symptom over the pulse or precedence of the pulse over the symptoms, the prescription must be justifiable. For that reason, the book, *Yi Fang Ji Jie (The Collected Annotations on Medical Formulas)*, really deserves close grinding (*i.e.*, close analysis and study).

The pulses in the three positions on the left hand indicate the viscera of the heart, liver, and kidneys and the bowels of the small intestine, gallbladder, and urinary bladder. The viscera pertain to yin, while the bowels to yang. These are called three yin and three yang. The pulses in the three positions on the right hand indicate the viscera of the lungs, spleen, and life gate and bowels of the large intestine, stomach, and triple burner. To feel the pulse, one should have the nails of the second, third, and fourth fingers cut, for the tips of the fingers are most sensitive. When one puts the tips of the fingers vertically over the pulse, one will never fail to perceive the most fine (messages of) stirring or tranquility, vacuity and repletion of the pulse. If one feels the pulse with the three fingers placed flat, one may fail to perceive the fine and subtle (messages from) the pulse.

# Table of Contents

# Chapter Fourteen

## Chapter One
# Heart-imparting Rhymes
# on Pulse Examination

Four kinds of pulse are the key criteria in examination: the floating, deep, slow, and rapid. The floating and deep can be discerned by light and heavy pressure of the fingers (respectively). The slow and rapid may (respectively) become the moderate and the racing. This can be identified by (counting) respirations. If a pulse is floating but forceless, it is a vacuous one. If it is floating and forceful, this is surging. A pulse deep but forceless is a weak pulse. If it is slightly deep but forceful, it is a replete pulse. A pulse slow but forceful is taken as a slippery pulse. If it is slow and forceless, the pulse may be a moderate or choppy one.[1] If a pulse is rapid and forceful, this is tight or bowstring.[2] If it is rapid but forceless, it is a scallion-stalk pulse. A floating, slow pulse indicates vacuity in the exterior. A deep, slow pulse reveals extreme internal cold. A floating, rapid pulse is undoubtedly an indication of exterior heat, while a deep, rapid pulse shows intense internal heat. The above explanations are not derived from works by the ancients but a subtle knowledge attained through my heart.[3]

---

[1] A moderate pulse, from a pathological point of view, refers to a pulse which is slightly slow. A choppy pulse is fine and slow in addition to being rough. Therefore, Liu sees both of these pulses as types of slow pulses.

[2] Wiseman gives stringlike for *xian*. We prefer bowstring.

[3] Readers should compare these definitions with those given in Bob Flaws's *The Secret of Chinese Pulse Diagnosis*, Blue Poppy Press, Boulder 1996. Some of them appear idiosyncratic and not standard.

# Diseases Ruled by the Various Kinds of Pulse

The floating pulse reveals wind (or) vacuity, and the scallion-stalk pulse indicates loss of blood. A slippery pulse indicates counterflow vomiting, while a replete one indicates heat. The bowstring pulse reveals hypertonicity, and a tight one indicates pain. If the pulse is surging, there is usually fever.

A deep pulse is an indication of cold accumulation pain, and a faint one reveals cold binding. The moderate pulse rules wind vacuity, and the choppy one indicates shortage of blood. A slow pulse indicates disease of obstinate cold, and a hidden one suggests assault by accumulation. The soggy and weak pulses are a little different, (respectively) revealing shortage of qi and blood.[4]

A long pulse reveals vigorous fever, and a short one points to food (accumulation). A vacuous pulse is, in general, an indication of abstraction of the mind. A skipping pulse[5] is a result of attacking gathering and accumulation and heat. A bound pulse reveals yin cold accumulation. A stirring pulse is an indication of fright palpitations, blood flooding, and strangury. The confined pulse[6] reveals cold pain (caused by) wood overwhelming the spleen. The regularly interrupted pulse shows soaring away of the righteous qi. The thin pulse is an indication of extremely desiccated essence and emaciated physical body.

---

[4] In most cases, the soggy pulse shows dampness and vacuity of blood, while the weak pulse reveals qi vacuity.

[5] A pulse is called skipping if it is rapid with occasional interruption. However, a racing, forceful pulse is also called skipping according to some authors.

[6] A confined pulse is a deep pulse which is long and replete as well as a little bowstring.

# Chapter Two
# General Essentials of Pulse Examination

The significance and the mechanisms of the pulse are extremely subtle and fine but can be clearly imparted to the heart (*i.e.*, mind) through examination. The heart pulse in the left inch (position) should be floating, large, and dissipated. The liver-gallbladder pulse in the left bar should be long and bowstring. The lung pulse in the right inch should be floating, choppy, and short. The spleen-stomach pulse in the right bar should be simultaneously moderate and large. The cubit pulse on both hands which is ascribed to the kidneys is expected to be deep and soft. All this indicates a healthy body free from disease.

The spring pulse is bowstring, and the summer pulse hooklike.[1] The autumn pulse is hairlike[2], and the winter pulse stonelike.[3] Congruence of the pulse with the seasons is a favorable (condition), while incongruence is unfavorable. The fingers should try to make a definite distinction between the generator and the restrainer.[4]

---

[1] A hooklike pulse is a surging pulse which is effulgent in coming but debilitated in retreating.

[2] A hairlike pulse is a floating and soft pulse. Some people describe it as a floating and choppy pulse.

[3] Stonelike is an epithet meaning deep, hard, and slippery.

[4] This refers to a relationship between the pulse images. In spring, which is wood, for example, if the pulse presents the autumn pulse, *i.e.*, a hairlike pulse, this is metal overwhelming or restraining wood, a very serious condition. Autumn is analogous to metal. If a hairlike pulse appears in winter when one expects to see a stonelike pulse, then this is mother metal generating child water. This is a vacuity disease.

3

Whenever the pulse in the human prognosis[5] on the left hand is exuberant, there are pathoconditions of wind, cold, summerheat, or dampness invariably with fever and aversion to cold. There are four kinds of pulses corresponding to these four pathoconditions. One must make a sure identification of them. If the pulse is floating but forceless, there is wind damage. If the pulse is floating and forceful, there is a cold damage condition. If the pulse is floating but vacuous, summerheat has damaged the heart. If the pulse is floating but moderate, there is damp disease. (In treating these,) one should guard against confusing effusion, dissipation, percolation and disinhibition, and, to protect the original destiny (*i.e.*, life), one should use harmonious and balanced medicinals.

Whenever the pulse in the qi opening[6] on the right hand is exuberant, there is an internal damage condition done by food and drink. Internal damage done by taxation and fatigue exhibits a floating, surging pulse. If food and drink damage the spleen, the pulse is surging and exuberant. There may also be involvement of the seven affects. Joy exhibits a dissipated pulse, and anger, a bowstring one, while anxiety manifests a choppy (pulse). Sorrow is revealed by a tight pulse, and thought by a bound one, while fear exhibits a deep (pulse). In case of fright, the pulse comes stirring and unsteady. To protect and quiet the whole, one should calm the stomach qi, but replenishing repletion and evacuating vacuity is able to cause detriment to one's destiny.

If the pulse is replete in the left bar, the liver has a surplus. If the pulse is choppy in the right bar, spleen earth is vacuous. A choppy pulse in the left bar indicates that the blood is insufficient. A slippery pulse in the right bar reveals the existence of food accumulation. A floating, scallion-stalk pulse in the left cubit is an indication of hematuria. A floating, surging pulse in the right cubit is a revelation of bound stools. If the pulse

---

[5] On the left hand, the position of the *cun* or inch or vessel opening is called the human prognosis (*ren ying*). One should note that the pulse at the Adam's apple is also called human prognosis (*ren ying*).

[6] On the right hand, the inch position is named the qi opening (*cun kou*).

is slow in the left cubit, yang affairs (*i.e.*, sexual performance) are debilitated. If the pulse is rapid in the right cubit, ministerial fire[7] is harsh.

(A pulse) arriving four times per respiration is a harmonious, calm or level (*i.e.*, normal pulse). Increase by one time indicates no great trouble. (A pulse) arriving three times (per respiration) is slow, while one arriving one or two times indicates collapse. (A pulse) arriving once per two respirations points to death. (A pulse) arriving six times (per respiration) is a rapid pulse, while (one) arriving seven times is beyond measure. (A pulse arriving) eight times suggests desertion. (A pulse arriving) nine times is a critical (condition), and ten times is dangerous.

If the pulse is absent from the upper and the lower[8], then yin and yang have expired. If the pulse is observed to have stopped coming and going, the original root is withered and exhausted. If the pulse is frequently interrupted, death will come before long; one need not hesitate to make this decision. In examining the pulse, one should count the respirations. If there is not one interruption in 50 beats, the body is free of disease. If prosperous life signs are felt under the fingers, (the patient) can rest reassured even though there is disease.

---

[7] Ministerial fire is kidney yang or life gate fire. Here, however, it refers to excessive sexual desire.

[8] The upper is the inch position or the vessel opening, while the lower is the cubit position.

# Chapter Three
# The Six Methods of Pulse Examination

When one puts down the fingers to feel the pulse, first of all one should focus one's attention on the heart (pulse). If the heart pulse is floating and large, this is the right shape. If it is floating and forceful, there is heat in the heart channel. The heat rules a festering tongue and pain in voiding urine. When there is common cold and wind cold, the pulse is bowstring and tight as well. If there is headache and fever and chills, the pulse is rapid. This is a little difficult to relieve. Fright palpitations and fearful throbbing exhibit a deep, thin, and weak pulse. If there is amassed heat in the upper burner, its response is a surging, large pulse.

Next, one should focus one's attention on the liver pulse. If it is bowstring and long, there is no bad consequence even though there is disease. If it suddenly becomes floating and large, there is wind making trouble. If it is surging and tight as well, there ought to be malaria or dysentery. A faint or a choppy (liver pulse) indicates shortage of yin blood. A rapid one is a result of anger, while a moderate one, of emaciation. Superabundant (pulse qi) is due to repletion, making known liver fire. If (the liver pulse) is deep and thin, as a rule there is vacuity.

As long as the kidney pulse feels deep, there is no disease. If it is surging and large, this shows that yin fire is generated. In males, if it is faint, the lower origin is insufficient. If it is slippery in females, pregnancy can be determined. If it is bowstring and tight, there is extreme vacuity. If it is scallion-stalk, there is precipitation of blood. If there is pain in the lumbus radiating to the rib-side, the pulse will appear to be slightly deep.

7

Vexatious heat in the five hearts[1] exhibits a surging yet forceless (kidney pulse). The offence of sexual taxation makes (the pulse) rapid and disquiet.

If, on examination, the pulse feels floating, short, and choppy in the right inch (position), the lungs are clean of disease. If evil qi surges up to give rise to frequent coughing, one should make a careful study (of the lung pulse) which ought to be surging and large. If the pulse is bowstring and tight, the throat is invariably dry and festering. When it is rapid, there is heat in the chest which makes one restless. If it is floating and forceful, there is external contraction of wind. A deep (lung) pulse rules welling abscess, and a slippery one indicates phlehm.

The spleen is of a dry nature and inclined to exhibit a slow (or) moderate pulse. When its pulse is slippery and rapid, food damage is made known. If it is surging and large, there is intense stomach fire. If it is bowstring and tight, there must be the disease of malaria. If it is vacuous and floating, there is diarrhea with an inflated abdomen. Belching and acid regurgitation are indicated by a rapid pulse; they are due to heat. When earth is unable to restrain water, the limbs will sustain puffy swelling. Then the kidney pulse, a deep, thin and faint pulse, will appear (instead).

Ministerial fire of the life gate is compatible with nothing but a still (*i.e.*, tranquil pulse).[2] Even though the pulse is deep and fine, there is no disease. On the contrary, if it is exuberant and effulgent, there is disastrous yin vacuity with night sweats and markedly wasted muscles (*i.e.*, flesh). If it is floating and surging, there is retching of blood and dream emission. If it is slippery and rapid, there is the pathocondition of clouded, flowery (*i.e.*, blurred) vision and deafness. If it is slow and moderate, this is usually a result of cold in the lower part (of the body). If it is effulgent in females, there ought to be pregnancy. [The life gate pulse.][3]

---

[1]  The five hearts refer to the palms, the soles of the feet, and the cardiac region.

[2]  Since the main pathology of ministerial fire is its stirring and stirring is the opposite of stillness, this line may also be read in a broader context. It is appropriate for ministerial fire to be nothing but still.

[3]  On the left hand, the promixal or cubit position is ascribed to the kidneys, while on the right hand, it is governed by the life gate.

## Chapter Four
# Poem on the Study of the Three Positions as a Whole

If the pulse is floating in all three positions, there is lung visceral wind[1] with aversion to cold, fever, and nasal congestion. If it is deep and slow, there is cold accumulation, and the true origin is exhausted. If it is bowstring and rapid, this reveals frenzy due to seething anger. If it is tight on both hands, there is cold and food (accumulation). If it is moderate in both bars, there is impediment and dribbling block. If it is vacuous, soggy, faint, and choppy, yin and yang are both exhausted. If it is surging and slippery, this is met in unbearable enduring diseases.

## Chapter Five
# The Necessity of Rational Inquiry

It is necessary to ask sick persons about their predilections. If inquiry acertains a heat disease, then it is appropriate to use cold (medicinals). If inquiry acertains a cold disease, then it is appropriate to use hot (medicinals). There are sick persons, who are confined to a secluded room, behind the drapes, or even have their heads covered up with quilts. They refuse to talk of their disease but ask the physician to make a diagnosis. If asked about the causes and origins (of their diseases) in some detail, they will say the (attending) physician is not qualified. If one is not

---

[1] This is commonly known as lung wind. Its pathogen is wind and it occurs in autumn, manifesting as copious sweating, aversion to cold, a pale face, occasional cough, shortness of breath, and relief during the day but exacerbation at night.

allowed to make a study of the physical form and complexion or sound and voice, or to inquire about the condition, but (is only allowed) to feel the pulse, it is a masterly physician who can determine death and life for the hundreds of diseases.

Therefore, a doctor should take time to ask (patients) what things they feel bitter about (*i.e.,* dislike), what things they miss, what things they desire, and what things they suspect (have done harm to them) and ask about their age and the thinness and fatness of their physical form. The doctor should ask how their diet and lifestyle are, whether their urination and defecation are inhibited or uninhibited, how their disease was at the onset and how it is now, how many days their disease has lasted, and what medicinals they have taken. If they are women, married or unmarried, it is necessary to ask about their menstruation. Postpartum, it is necessary to ask whether there is a lochia and what its amount is. If a small child suffers from abhorrence of cold and vigorous fever, it is necessary to ask whether maculopapules (*i.e.,* pox, such as measles) have already erupted.

In regard to the various diseases with pain, it is necessary to ask whether there have been knocks or falls.

The above is the great method (of inquiry). One must by all means make a careful inquiry about everything. One should correlate one's own observation with the account (of the patient). They may agree or disagree. Then one should take both into consideration. This way a sure-fire success will be accomplished.

# Chapter Six
# Channel Conducting Medicinals

*G*ao Ben (Radix Et Rhizoma Ligustici Chinensis) and *Qiang Huo* (Radix Et Rhizoma Notopterygii) are able to move along the hand and foot *tai yang* channels. *Chai Hu* (Radix Bupleuri) is always used as usher to the destination of the *shao yang* and *jue yin*. The hand and foot *yang ming* require *Bai Zhi* (Radix Angelicae Dahuricae), *Sheng Ma* (Rhizoma Cimicifugae), and *Ge Gen* (Radix Puerariae). For the lungs, use *Bai Zhi* (Radix Angelicae Dahuricae), *Sheng Ma* (Rhizoma Cimicifugae), and *Cong Bai* (Bulbus Allii Fistulosi). The spleen responds to *Sheng Ma* (Rhizoma Cimicifugae) and *Bai Shao* (Radix Albus Paeoniae Lactiflorae). As for the heart channel, *Huang Lian* (Rhizoma Coptidis Chinensis) is the envoy. For the kidneys, only adding *Gui Zhi* (Ramulus Cinnamomi Cassiae) is magical. If these medicinals are prescribed in accordance with the channels, one will cure diseases as if having consulted the gods.

# Chapter Seven
# Prose & Verse Transmitting the Heart of Using Medicinals

*T*he subtlety in prescribing medicinals is like that of commanding an army. What is decisive is not the amounts of armies but putting them to their best use. In (prescribing) medicinals, what is vital is not variety but the choice of what is effective. One should bear in mind that *Huang Lian*(Rhizoma Coptidis Chinensis) clears the heart channel of visiting fire, and that *Huang Bai* (Cortex Phellodendri) downbears wandering ministerial fire. *Huang Qin* (Radix Scutellariae Baicalensis) is most wonderful in draining lung fire, while *Zhi Zi* (Fructus Gardeniae Jasminoidis) clears stomach heat magically. *Mang Xiao* (Mirabilitum) frees the flow of the stools when they are dry and bound. *Da Huang* (Radix Et Rhizoma Rhei) is the general (competent in) flushing.[1] *Xi Jiao* (Cornu Rhinocerotis) resolves heart heat. *Niu Huang* (Calculus Bovis) settles gallbladder fright.[2] *Lian Qiao* (Fructus Forsythiae Suspensae) drains the six channels of fire. *Ju Hua* (Flos Chrysanthemi Morifolii) brightens clouded eyes. *Hua Shi* (Talcum) disinhibits blocked or inhibited urination. *Shi Gao* (Gypsum Fibrosum) drains upflaming and steaming stomach fire. *Shan Dou Gen* (Radix Sophorae Subprostratae) resolves heat toxins to treat throat impediment. *Sang Bai Pi* (Cortex Radicis Mori Albi) drains evils from the lungs, disinhibiting collecting water. *Long Dan* (Radix Gentianae Scabrae) treats heat in the liver. *Qu Mai* (Herba Dianthi) disinhibits the urinary bladder when it causes strangury. *Bie Jia* (Carapax Amydae Sinensis) treats malaria as well as aggregation. *Gui Ban* (Plastrum Testudinis) supplements yin and hence the heart. *Yin Chen* (Herba Artemisiae Capillaris) treats jaundice and disinhibits water. *Xiang Ru* (Herba Elsholtziae Seu Moslae) treats sudden turmoil (*i.e.,* choleraic disease) to clear the chest. *Chai Hu* (Radix Bupleuri) abates alternating cold and heat. *Qian Hu* (Radix Peucedani) treats phlegm ascent cough. *Yuan Shen* (Radix Scrophulariae Ningpoensis) treats bound toxin abscesses and flat abscesses, clearing and disinhibiting the throat and diaphragm. *Sha Shen* (Radix Glehniae Littoralis) supplements yin vacuity causing cough to protect the lung channel. *Zhu Ye* (Folium Bambusae) and *Zhu Ru* (Caulis Bambusae In Taeniis) treat vacuity vexation effectively. *Mao Gen* (Rhizoma Imperatae Cylindricae) and *Ou Jie* (Nodus Rhizomatis Nelumbinis Nuciferae) arrest vomiting and stop nosebleeding usually with remarkable results. *Ku Shen* (Radix Sophorae Flavescentis) treats mania and welling abscesses. *Di Yu* (Radix Sanguisorbae Officinalis) relieves bloody dysentery and checks blood flooding. *Che Qian Zi* (Semen Plantaginis) disinhibits water to stop diarrhea. *Gua Lou Ren* (Semen Trichosanthis Kirlowii) downbears phlegm to clear the chest. *Qin Jiao* (Radix Gentianae Macrophyllae) eliminates steaming bones with taxation

---

[1] General (*Jun*) is another name of *Da Huang* (Radix Et Rhizoma Rhei). This name implies that *Da Huang* is a very drastic medicinal, very good at precipitating from the intestines what is gathered or accumulated.

[2] Actually, this is simply fright. Because the gallbladder governs decision-making, liability to fright, irresoluteness, and timidity are all impugned to the gallbladder.

heat. *Dan Pi* (Cortex Radicis Moutan) breaks up blood accumulation to move menstrual flow. *Shu Di* (cooked Radix Rehmanniae) supplements the blood and treats detriment. *Sheng Di* (uncooked Radix Rehmanniae) cools the blood to enrich yin. *Bai Shao* (Radix Albus Paeoniae Lactiflorae) treats abdominal pain, and, because it is able to supplement and astringe as well, it also eliminates vexatious heat from the upper part (of the body). *Chi Shao* (Radix Rubrus Paeoniae Lactiflorae) frees the flow of blood stasis, and, because it is able to disperse and drain as well, it also disinhibits the lower abdomen. *Mai Dong* (Tuber Ophiopogonis Japonici) engenders the pulse to clear the heart and suppresses coughing above. *Tian Dong* (Tuber Asparagi Cochinensis) disperses phlegm and moistens the lungs, penetrating the kidney channel below. *Di Gu Pi* (Cortex Radicis Lycii Chinensis) treats consumptive steaming bones with heat arising in the night. *Zhi Mu* (Rhizoma Anemarrhenae Asphodeloidis) abates blazing fire in the kidney channel. *Ge Gen* (Radix Puerariae) quenches thirst and resolves the muscles. *Ze Xie* (Rhizoma Alismatis) supplements yin and is able to percolate and disinhibit. The above are medicinals of cold nature. Before prescribing them, one should weigh prudently.

It should be understood that hot medicinals may warm the channels. *Ma Huang* (Herba Ephedrae) exteriorizes cold evils by promoting perspiration. *Guan Gui* (tubiform Cortex Cinnamomi Cassiae) treats invading cold qi. *Mu Xiang* (Radix Auklandiae Lappae) regulates the qi to treat abdominal pain. *Chen Xiang* (Lignum Aquilariae Agallochae) downbears the qi and treats lumbago. *Ding Xiang* (Flos Caryophylli) arrests retching, and warms stomach cold. *Huo Xiang* (Herba Agastachis Seu Pogostemi) arrests vomiting and invigorates the stomach duct by warming it. *Wu Zhu Yu* (Fructus Evodiae Rutecarpae) penetrates the lower abdomen to treat its cold pain. *Shan Zhu Yu* (Fructus Corni Officinalis) strengthens the lumbus and kidneys to astringe essence. *Dou Kou* (Fructus Alpiniae Katsumadae) and *Sha Ren* (Fructus Amomi) rectify the qi and food (accumulation) in the chest. *Fu Pi* (Pericarpium Arecae Catechu) and *Hou Po* (Cortex Magnoliae Officinalis) treat abdominal inflation. *Bai Dou Kou* (Fructus Cardamomi) opens the stomach and eliminates stagnant (food). *Yuan Hu Suo* (Rhizoma Corydalis Yanhusuo) treats the qi and blood and regulates menstruation as well. *Fu Zi* (Radix Lateralis Praeparatus Aconiti Carmichaeli) is a medicinal to recover yang and relieve yin cold. *Gan Jiang*

13

(dry Rhizoma Zingiberis) treats cold and is able to turn the viscera and bowels warm. *Cao Guo* (Fructus Amomi Tsao-ko) disperses and dissolves abiding food. *Bing Lang* (Semen Arecae Catechu) removes accumulations and pushes out the stale. *Cong Rong* (Herba Cistanchis Deserticolae) invigorates yang to secure the root. *Lu Rong* (Cornu Parvum Cervi) boosts the kidneys and engenders essence. *Suo Yang Tzi* (Herba Cynomorii Songarici) is a medicinal most able to check seminal leaking. *Tu Si Zi* (Semen Cuscutae Chinensis) tends to secure the heavenly true. *Mo Yao* (Resina Myrrhae) and *Ru Xiang* (Resina Olibani) dissipate congealed blood to relieve pain. *Er Chou* (Semen Pharbiditis) and *Ba Dou* (Semen Crotonis Tiglii), which clash with one another, precipitate accumulation to resolve fecal block. *Zi Su* (Folium Perillae Frutescentis) dissipates wind cold, and *Su Zi* (Fructus Perillae Frutescentis) is able to downbear the qi. *Chuan Jiao* (Pericarpium Zanthoxyli Bungeani) abates roundworm reversal, and its seeds treat (qi) ascent panting. *Wu Ling Zhi* (Feces Trogopterori Seu Pteromi) treats blood pain in the heart and abdomen. *Da Hui Xiang* (Fructus Illicii Veri) treats qi pain in the small intestine. These are the indications of hot medicinals, which should be prescribed in the capacity of sovereign, minister, assistant, or envoy.

When speaking of warm medicinals, one should put their abilities to their best use. *Gan Cao* (Radix Glycyrrhizae) is the senior state minister in terms of harmonizing the center. *Ren Shen* (Radix Panacis Ginseng) is an arch god of supplementing qi. *Ting Li* (Semen Lepidii Seu Descurainiae) downbears lung panting and disinhibits water, but it is classified into two species, the sweet and the bitter.[3] *Fu Ling* (Sclerotium Poriae Cocos) supplements spleen vacuity and is able to disinhibit and percolate, but one should distinguish between the red and the white.[4] *Huang Qi* (Radix Astragali Membranacei) supplements the defensive to check sweating.

---

[3] *Ting Li* (Semen Lepidii Seu Descurainiae) may taste sweet or bitter and, therefore, is divided into two sub-species. The sweet is temperate in precipitating water, while the bitter is drastic.

[4] *Fu Ling* (Sclerotium Poriae Cocos) is a bland and balanced flavored medicinal proving to be mild in both qi and flavor. The red, which is *Chi Fu Ling* (Sclerotium Rubrum Poriae Cocos), is somewhat disinhibiting, while the white, *Bai Fu Ling* (Sclerotium [Album] Poriae Cocos), is somewhat supplementing.

*Shan Yao* (Radix Dioscoreae Oppositae) boosts the kidneys and opens the heart. *E Zhu* (Rhizoma Curcumae Zedoariae) and *San Leng* (Rhizoma Sparganii) disperse lump glomus developing from hard accumulation. *Mai Ya* (Fructus Germinatus Hordei Vulgaris) and *Shen Qu* (Massa Medica Fermentata) disperse food and drink to loosen inflation (*i.e.*, distention). To normalize the qi and transform phlegm, *Chen Pi* (Pericarpium Citri Reticulatae) can be used. To loosen the center and relieve the diaphragm, *Zhi Ke* (Fructus Citri Aurantii) should be employed. *Bai Zhu* (Rhizoma Atractylodis Macrocephalae) fortifies the spleen and eliminates dampness. *Dang Gui* (Radix Angelicae Sinensis) supplements blood and regulates menstruation. *Ban Xia* (Rhizoma Pinelliae Ternatae) treats phlegm and dries the stomach. *Zhi Shi* (Fructus Immaturus Citri Aurantii) removes accumulations and pushes out the stale. *Chuan Xiong* (Radix Ligustici Wallichii) is an important medicinal for treating headache. *Tao Ren* (Semen Pruni Persicae) is precious as a pearl when used to break blood stasis. *Ai Ye* (Foluim Artemisiae Argyii) quiets the fetus and treats flooding and spotting. *Xiang Fu* (Rhizoma Cyperi Rotundi) normalizes the qi and regulates the channels[5] as well. *Xing Ren* (Semen Pruni Armeniacae) suppresses wind cold coughing. *Wu Wei* (Fructus Schisandrae Chinensis) astringes ascending lung qi. *Fang Feng* (Radix Ledebouriellae Divaricatae) is an indispensable medicinal for various wind (diseases). *Jing Jie* (Herba Schizonepetae Tenuifoliae) clears the head and eyes, and cures (blood) flooding. *Shan Zha* (Fructus Crataegi) disperses meat food accumulation. *Xi Xin* (Herba Asari Cum Radice) relieves *shao yin* headache. *Zi Wei Hua* (Flos Campsitis Grandiflorae) frees the channels (*i.e.*, menses) and induces abortion. *Suan Zao Ren* (Semen Zizyphi Spinosae) constrains sweating and calms the spirit. *Gao Ben* (Radix Et Rhizoma Ligustici Chinensis) relieves aching on the top of the head. *Jie Geng* (Radix Platycodi Grandiflori) is able to carry (other) medicinals like a boat. *Du Zhong* (Cortex Eucommiae Ulmoidis) strengthens the lumbus and knees and supplements the kidneys. *Hong Hua* (Flos Carthami Tinctorii) resuscitates blood dizziness and frees the flow of the channels. The above are the natures and qi of warm medicinals. Students should go by (the prescriptions).

---

[5] The word channel or *jing* in this case refers to menstruation. In this case, it is an abbereviation for *yue jing* or menstruatrion.

Since three kinds of medicinals are now clear, next it is time to enumerate the balancing. *Chang Shan* (Radix Dichroae Febrifugae) is used to interrupt malaria. *A Wei* (Resina Ferulae Asafoetidae) is used to disperse concretions. *Fang Ji* (Radix Stephaniae Tetrandrae) and *Mu Gua* (Fructus Chaenomlis Lagenariae) eliminate dampness swelling from the lower burner. *Chang Pu* (Rhizoma Acori Graminei) and *Yuan Zhi* (Radix Polygalae Tenuifoliae) free the spirit light of the heart and abdomen.[6] To strengthen the lumbus and knees, nothing is better than *Hu Gu* (Os Trigridis). To settle fright palpitations, *Fu Shen* (Sclerotium Pararadicis Poriae Cocos) ought to be used. *E Jiao* (Gelatinum Corii Asini) suppresses coughing and staunches bleeding. *Mu Li* (Concha Ostreae) astringes sweating and essence. *Qiang Huo* (Radix Et Rhizoma Notopterygii) dissipates wind to relieve aching in the bone joints. *Dong Hua* (Flos Tussilaginis Farfarae) suppresses coughing and downbears ascending lung fire. *Du Huo* (Radix Angelicae Pubescentis) and *Ji Sheng* (Ramulus Loranthi Seu Visci) are able to cope with wind dampness in the foot and knee. *Bo He* (Herba Menthae Haplocalysis) and *Bai Zhi* (Radix Angelicae Dahuricae) dissipate wind aching in the forehead. *Mu Zei* (Herba Equiseti Hiemalis) and *Ji Li* (Fructus Tribuli Terrestris) abate floating screens in the eye. *Yuan Ming Fen* (Mirabilitum Depuratum) and *Hai Fen* (Ovum Notarchi Leachii Freeri) downbear soaring phlegm fire. *Qing Pi* (Pericarpium Citri Reticulatae Viride) quells wood, and *Zi Wan* (Radix Asteris Tatarici) restrains metal. *Wu Jia Pi* (Cortex Radicis Acanthopanacis) disperses swelling and quickens the blood. *Tian Hua Fen* (Radix Trichosanthis Kirlowii) quenches thirst and engenders fluids. *Niu Bang Zi* (Fructus Arctii Lappae) clears and disinhibits the throat. *Yi Yi Ren* (Semen Coicis Lachryma-jobi) rectifies foot qi[7] causing difficult walking. *Hu Po* (Succinum) quiets the spirit and disinhibits water. *Zhu Sha* (Cinnabar) settles the heart and stabilizes fright. *Bei Mu* (Bulbus Fritillariae) opens the depression of the heart and chest and, hence, treats bound phlegm. *Bai*

---

[6] This sentence implies that the two medicinals can cure problems involving the chest and abdomen, such as pain, distention, and oppression, and resolve some mental disorders (*viz.* spirit light), such as fainting, impaired memory, and epilepsy.

[7] This is also known as slackening wind or foot weakness. It is a syndrome of swelling and numbness of the lower limbs complicated by cardiac troubles and some mental disorders.

*He* (Bulbus Lilii) rectifies vacuity taxation coughing and, in addition, treats *gu* toxins.[8] *Sheng Ma* (Rhizoma Cimicifugae) raises the qi and dissipates wind. *Niu Xi* (Radix Achyranthis Bidentatae) tends to descend to strengthen the bones. To disinhibit water, it is necessary to use *Zhu Ling* (Sclerotium Polypori Umbellati). To dry dampness, *Cang Zhu* (Rhizoma Atractylodis) is the right choice. *Gou Qi Zi* (Fructus Lycii Chinensis) brightens the eyes and engenders essence. *Lu Jiao Jiao* (Gelatinum Cornu Cervi) supplements vacuity with great results. *Tian Ma* (Rhizoma Gastrodiae Elatae) treats all wind with shaking and dizzy vision. *Mu Tong* (Caulis Akebiae) treats difficult and inhibited urination. *Tian Nan Xing* (Rhizoma Arsiaematis) is most able to treat wind phlegm. *Lai Fu Zi* (Semen Raphani Sativi) is particularly able to cure flour food (accumulation).

The above is an outline of medicinal natures. One should get it by heart as a secret art.

---

[8]  *Gu* toxins refer to a sudden, often infectious condition of diverse manifestations believed to be caused by toxic worms or insects.

## Chapter Eight
# Rhymes on the Ruling Medicinals (Used) in Treating Disease

Headache necessitates the use of *Chuan Xiong* (Radix Ligustici Wallichii). If it fails to effect a cure, add appropriate channel conductors. For the *tai yang*, add *Qiang Huo* (Radix Et Rhizoma Notopterygii) and a little *Chai Hu* (Radix Bupleuri). For the *yang ming*, it is necessary to prescribe *Bai Zhi* (Radix Angelicae Dahuricae). For the *tai yin*, add *Cang Zhu* (Rhizoma Atractylodis) and a little *Xi Xin* (Herba Asari Cum Radice). In case of the *jue yin*, using *Wu Zhu Yu* (Fructus Evodiae Rutecarpae) is never a mistake. Pain in the top of the head may differ from person to person; it requires use of *Gao Ben* (Radix Et Rhizoma Ligustici Chinensis) in place of *Chuan Xiong* (Radix Ligustici Wallichii).

For pain in the limbs, it is necessary to use *Qiang Huo* (Radix Et Rhizoma Notopterygii), which is also credited with the ability to eliminate not only wind but dampness. To treat lower abdominal pain, one should use *Qing Pi* (Pericarpium Citri Reticulatae Viride). Glomus below the heart calls for *Huang Lian* (Rhizoma Coptidis Chinensis) and *Zhi Shi* (Fructus Immaturus Citri Aurantii). Abdominal pain requires using *Bai Shao Yao* (Radix Albus Paeoniae Lactiflorae). If it is due to cold, add *Rou Gui* (Cortex Cinnamomi Cassiae). If it is due to heat, add *Huang Bai* (Cortex Phellodendri). For narrowing of the abdomen[1], *Cang Zhu* (Rhizoma Atractylodis) is appropriate. For abdominal distention and inflation, use ginger (mix-fried) *Hou Po* (Cortex Magnoliae Officinalis). Among those that are used to treat replete heat in the abdomen, *Da Huang* (Radix Et Rhizoma Rhei) and *Mang Xiao* (Mirabilitum) have the most effective action. For vacuity

---

[1] Narrowing of the abdomen implies abdominal distention, gripping pain, food accumulation, etc.

**19**

heat and vacuity sweating, use *Huang Qi* (Radix Astragali Membranacei). For floating heat in the skin, *Huang Qin* (Radix Scutellariae Baicalensis) is an appropriate medicinal. For aching and pain in the rib-side, intermittent fever, and late afternoon tidal fever, *Chai Hu* (Radix Bupleuri) is an appropriate medicinal.

When the spleen and stomach are affected by dampness, there will be a lack of strength, fatigue, and somnolence. For this, use *Bai Zhu* (Rhizoma Atractylodis Macrocephalae). For swelling due to dampness combined with fire evils in the lower burner, use *Zhi Mu* (Rhizoma Anemarrhenae Asphodeloidis), *Fang Ji* (Radix Stephaniae Tetrandrae), *Long Dan* (Radix Gentianae Scabrae), and wine (mix-fried) *Huang Bai* (Cortex Phellodendri). For damp heat in the upper burner, use *Huang Qin* (Radix Scutellariae Baicalensis). Damp heat in the middle burner can be resolved by *Huang Lian* (Rhizoma Coptidis Chinensis).

To quench thirst, use *Gan Ge* (dry Radix Puerariae) and *Tian Hua Fen* (Radix Trichosanthis Kirlowii). *Ban Xia* (Rhizoma Pinelliae Ternatae) dries the spleen, but is prohibited in thirst. Cough requires using *Wu Wei Zi* (Fructus Schisandrae Chinensis), while panting requires *E Jiao* (Gelatinum Corii Asini). *Zhi Shi* (Fructus Immaturus Citri Aurantii) and *Huang Lian* (Rhizoma Coptidis Chinensis) treat abiding food. Vexatious heat in the chest requires *Zhi Zi Ren* (Fructus Gardeniae Jasminoidis). Watery diarrhea requires *Shao Yao* (Radix Paeoniae Lactiflorae), *Fu Ling* (Sclerotium Poriae Cocos) and *Bai Zhu* (Rhizoma Atractylodis Macrocephalae).

To regulate the qi, it is necessary to use *Mu Xiang* (Radix Auklandiae Lappae). It is, however, not good when there is exuberant qi.[2] To supplement the qi, it is necessary to use *Ren Shen* (Radix Panacis Ginseng). However, this is not an appropriate medicinal when there is heat in the lung channel. When phlegm drool causes disease, *Ban Xia* (Rhizoma Pinelliae Ternatae) is required. If there is heat, add *Huang Qin* (Radix Scutellariae Baicalensis); if there is wind, add *Nan Xing* (Rhizoma Arisaematis). When cold phlegm causes glomus blockage in the chest, two

---

[2] *Mu Xiang* (Radix Auklandiae Lappae) is a very good medicinal for any sort of qi problem, including qi exuberance. The author may mean that its use is prohibited when there is exuberant heat.

materials, *Bai Zhu* (Rhizoma Atractylodis Macrocephalae) and *Chen Pi* (Pericarpium Citri Reticulatae), should be added. For pain in the stomach duct, use *Cao Dou Kou* (Semen Alpiniae Katsumadai). If this is mixed with heat, *Huang Qin* (Radix Scutellariae Baicalensis) and *Huang Lian* (Rhizoma Coptidis Chinensis) should be used together.

For eye pain, use *Huang Lian* (Rhizoma Coptidis Chinensis) and *Dang Gui Gen* (Radix Angelicae Sinensis). For fright palpitation and abstraction, use *Fu Shen* (Sclerotium Pararadicis Poriae Cocos). When urine turns yellowish, use *Huang Bai* (Cortex Phellodendri). When urination is difficult, the addition of *Ze Xie* (Rhizoma Alismatis) works wonders. For qi pricking pains[3], *Zhi Ke* (Fructus Citri Aurantii) is required. For blood pain, *Dang Gui* (Radix Angelicae Sinensis) is used, but one should divide (*i.e.*, discriminate) above and below.[4] Dysentery is treated with *Dang Gui* (Radix Angelicae Sinensis) and *Bai Shao* (Radix Albus Paeoniae Lactiflorae). (To treat) malaria, *Chai Hu* (Radix Bupleuri) is the sovereign (ingredient). Blood stagnation requires *Tao Ren* (Semen Pruni Persicae) and *Su Mu* (Lignum Sappan). Qi stagnation requires *Qing Pi* (Pericarpium Citri Reticulatae Viride) and *Zhi Ke* (Fructus Citri Aurantii). (However,) if *Zhi Ke* (Fructus Citri Aurantii) and *Qing Pi* (Pericarpium Citri Reticulatae Viride) are used in large quantities, they will contrarily drain original qi and, therefore, should be reduced in amounts.

Whenever purely cold or purely hot medicinals are used, it is necessary to use *Gan Cao* (Radix Glycyrrhizae) to moderate their force. If cold and hot (medicinals) are used in combination, it also has to be employed to get rid of their attacking (actions) by balancing their natures. Center fullness, however, does not allow for taking sweet.[5] One has to take this into consideration in treatment.

---

[3] This refers to pain and itching in the skin caused by wind, dampness, and cold.

[4] *Dang Gui* (Radix Angelicae Sinensis) mainly treats blood disease, curing pain in the lower burner. But it also treats pain in the upper part of the body. When it is used to treat troubles in the upper body, headache for example, it should be processed with wine or some other medicinal which may carry it upward.

[5] *Gan Cao* (Radix Glycyrrhizae) means "sweet herb" in Chinese. Therefore, this sentence implies that *Gan Cao* is among the medicinals that are prohibited in case of center fullness. In a wider sense, however, any sweet medicinals are prohibited when treating center fullness.

# Chapter Nine
# Song on Additions & Subtractions
## to *Si Jun Zi Tang*

*S*i Jun (Four Gentlemen [Decoction]) is composed of *Ren Shen* (Radix Panacis Ginseng), *Bai Zhu* (Rhizoma Atractylodis Macrocephalae), *Fu Ling* (Sclerotium Poriae Cocos), and *Gan Cao* (Radix Glycyrrhizae). It is as precious as a jewel for supplementing the center and boosting the qi. When *Chen Pi* (Pericarpium Citri Reticulatae) is added, this formula is called *Yi Gong San* (Special Achievement Powder). For qi vacuity spontaneous sweating, it is good to add *Huang Qi* (Radix Astragali Membranacei). If *Ju Pi* (Pericarpium Citri Reticulatae) and *Ban Xia* (Rhizoma Pinelliae Ternatae) are added, this formula is called *Liu Jun [Zi] Tang* (Six Gentlemen Decoction), which is better than any other (formula) for fortifying the spleen and harmonizing the stomach. With *Xiang Fu* (Rhizoma Cyperi Rotundi) and *Sha Ren* (Fructus Amomi) (added) as a pair, it is able to disperse (abiding) food.[1] Retching and vomiting due to cold stomach requires *Ding Xiang* (Flos Caryophylli) and *Huo Xiang* (Herba Agastachis Seu Pogostemi) as envoys.[2]

---

[1]  This formula is called *Xiang Sha Liu Jun Tang* (Auklandia & Amomum Six Gentlemen Decoction).

[2]  Because this whole chapter focuses on *Si Jun Tang* (Four Gentlemen Decoction), all prescriptions in this chapter are based on this formula whether or not it is mentioned by name. In some instances, we have inserted the name of the formula for extra clarification. This is also the case with the following four chapters.

*Shi Quan* (Ten [Ingredients] Completely [& Greatly Supplementing Decoction]) includes *Si Wu* (Four Materials [Decoction])[3] and *Si Jun* (Four Gentlemen [Decoction]). These are boiled together with *Huang Qi* (Radix Astragali Membranacei), *Rou Gui* (Cortex Cinnamomi Cassiae), *Sheng Jiang* (uncooked Rhizoma Zingiberis) and *Da Zao* (Fructus Zizyphi Jujubae). This enriches the blood and qi and makes the spleen and stomach strong. It is the first choice for taxation damage as well as for vacuity and weakness.

*Yang Rong Tang* (Nourish the Constructive Decoction) is similar to *Shi Quan* (Ten [Ingredients] Completely [& Greatly Supplementing Decoction] in composition). It has *Wu Wei Zi* (Fructus Schisandrae Chinensis), *Yuan Zhi* (Radix Polygalae Tenuifoliae), and *Chen Pi* (Pericarpium Citri Reticulatae), but is without *Chuan Xiong* (Radix Ligustici Wallichii). This is for fatigue, emaciation, a pale facial complexion, and tidal (fever) with sweating. To combat dream emission, *Long Gu* (Os Draconis), *Mu Li* (Concha Ostreae), and *Lian Xu* (Stamen Nelumbinis Nuciferae) can be added.

Tidal fever with no sweating requires the addition of *Dang Gui* (Radix Angelicae Sinensis), *Bai Shao* (Radix Albus Paeoniae Lactiflorae), *Ban Xia* (Rhizoma Pinelliae Ternatae), *Chai Hu* (Radix Bupleuri), and powdered *Ge Gen* (Radix Puerariae) (to *Si Jun Zi Tang*).

For spontaneous sweating, add *Chen Pi* (Pericarpium Citri Reticulatae), *Huang Qi* (Radix Astragali Membranacei), *Shu Di* (cooked Radix Rehmanniae), *Dang Gui* (Radix Angelicae Sinensis), *Mu Li* (Concha Ostreae), *Wu Mei* (Fructus Pruni Mume), *Suan Zao* (Semen Zizyphi Spinosae), and *Bai Shao* (Radix Albus Paeoniae Lactiflorae).

If sweat appears nowhere but in the center of the chest, this indicates *Si Jun* (Four Gentlemen [Decoction]) expanded by *Chen Pi* (Pericarpium Citri

---

[3] *Si Wu Tang* (Four Materials Decoction) is composed of *Dang Gui* (Radix Angelicae Sinensis), *Di Huang* (Radix Rehmanniae), *Shao Yao* (Radix Paeoniae Lactiflorae), and *Chuan Xiong* (Radix Ligustici Wallichii).

Reticulatae), *Dang Gui* (Radix Angelicae Sinensis), and *Suan Zao* (Semen Zizyphi Spinosae) in addition to *Mai Dong* (Tuber Ophiopogonis Japonici), *Bai Shao* (Radix Albus Paeoniae Lactiflorae), mix-fried *Huang Lian* (Rhizoma Coptidis Chinensis), *Chen Sha* (Cinnabar), *Wu Mei* (Fructus Pruni Mume), and *Da Zao* (Fructus Zizyphi Jujubae).

Distressing taxation fatigue with no generalized fever can be stopped by (adding) *Mai Dong* (Tuber Ophiopogonis Japonici), *Wu Wei Zi* (Fructus Schisandrae Chinensis), *Chen Pi* (Pericarpium Citri Reticulatae), and *Huang Qi* (Radix Astragali Membranacei) to (Four Gentlemen Decoction) with *Fu Ling* (Sclerotium Poriae Cocos) subtracted.

For glomus and fullness with qi congestion and vacuity of the righteous qi, (this formula) should stand together with *Chen Pi* (Pericarpium Citri Reticulatae), *Dang Gui* (Radix Angelicae Sinensis), *Mu Xiang* (Radix Auklandiae Lappae), and *Sha Ren* (Fructus Amomi).

For forgetfulness, it is good (to add) *Huang Qi* (Radix Astragali Membranacei), *Yuan Zhi* (Radix Polygalae Tenuifoliae), *Mu Xiang* (Radix Auklandiae Lappae), *Chang Pu* (Rhizoma Acori Graminei), *Long Yan* (Arillus Euphoriae-Longanae), *Dang Gui* (Radix Angelicae Sinensis), and *Suan Zao* (Semen Zizyphi Spinosae).

For headache with vomiting of water, prescribe *Liu Jun Tang* (Six Gentlemen Decoction) plus *Dang Gui* (Radix Angelicae Sinensis), *Huang Qi* (Radix Astragali Membranacei), *Mu Xiang* (Radix Auklandiae Lappae), and *Pao Jiang* (blast-fried Rhizoma Zingiberis).

For qi vacuity with hasty breathing, shortness of breath, panting and no phlegm, tack on *Ren Shen* (Radix Panacis Ginseng), *Ju Hong* (Exocarpium Citri Erythrocarpae), *Sha Ren* (Fructus Amomi), and *Su Zi* (Fructus Perillae Frutescentis) along with *Sang Pi* (Cortex Radicis Mori Albi), *Dang Gui* (Radix Angelicae Sinensis), *Jiang* (Rhizoma Zingiberis), *Da Zao* (Fructus Zizyphi Jujubae), *Chen Xiang* (Lignum Aquilariae Agallochae), and water-ground *Mu Xiang* (Radix Auklandiae Lappae).

If, after relief of sudden turmoil (*i.e.*, choleraic disease), there arises headache with generalized aching complicated by a dry mouth, fever, and lack of strength of the limbs, add *Wu Wei* (Fructus Schisandrae Chinensis), *Dang Gui* (Radix Angelicae Sinensis), *Chai Hu* (Radix Bupleuri), *Bai Shao* (Radix Albus Paeoniae Lactiflorae), *Wu Mei* (Fructus Pruni Mume), *Zhi Zi* (Fructus Gardeniae Jasminoidis), *Mai Dong* (Tuber Ophiopogonis Japonici), and *Chen Pi* (Pericarpium Citri Reticulatae).

In case of generalized heaviness and aching complicated by somnolence, a bland taste in the mouth, aversion to cold, and frequent voidings of urine, to *Liu Jun* (Six Gentlemen [Decoction]), add *Bai Shao* (Radix Albus Paeoniae Lactiflorae), *Huang Lian* (Rhizoma Coptidis Chinensis), *Huang Qi* (Radix Astragali Membranacei), *Ze Xie* (Rhizoma Alismatis), *Chai Hu* (Radix Bupleuri), *Qiang Huo* (Radix Et Rhizoma Notopterygii), and *Du Huo* (Radix Angelicae Pubescentis).

For dizziness in fat persons, to *Liu Jun* (Six Gentlemen [Decoction]), add *Chuan Xiong* (Radix Ligustici Wallichii), *Dang Gui* (Radix Angelicae Sinensis), *Huang Qi* (Radix Astragali Membranacei), *Jie Geng* (Radix Platycodi Grandiflori), *Bai Zhi* (Radix Angelicae Dahuricae), and *Tian Ma* (Rhizoma Gastrodiae Elatae).

Turbid urine requires *Si Jun* (Four Gentlemen [Decoction]) plus *Yi Zhi* (Fructus Alpiniae Oxyphyllae), *Chen Pi* (Pericarpium Citri Reticulatae), *Huang Qi* (Radix Astragali Membranacei), *Shu Di* (cooked Radix Rehmanniae), *Dang Gui* (Radix Angelicae Sinensis), and *Sheng Ma* (Rhizoma Cimicifugae).

For glomus and fullness, append *Bing Lang* (Semen Arecae Catechu), *Zhi Shi* (Fructus Immaturus Citri Aurantii), and *Huang Lian* (Rhizoma Coptidis Chinensis).

In case of red eyes due to blood congestion, add *Long Dan* (Radix Gentianae Scabrae). In case of headache, add *Chuan Xiong* (Radix Ligustici Wallichii) and *Man Jing Zi* (Fructus Viticis). In case of diarrhea, decoct (Four Gentlemen Decoction) together with *Bai Shao* (Radix Albus

Paeoniae Lactiflorae), *Ze Xie* (Rhizoma Alismatis), and *Fu Ling* (Sclerotium Poriae Cocos).

For copious sweating, (adding) *Huang Qi* (Radix Astragali Membranacei), *Bai Zhu* (Rhizoma Atractylodis Macrocephalae), and *Gui Shen* (Corpus Radicis Angelicae Sinensis) is good. The following (formulas) cannot be short of them. For brain pain, add *Gao Ben* (Radix Et Rhizoma Ligustici Chinensis) and *Xi Xin* (Herba Asari Cum Radice). For frontal headache, add *Sheng Ma* (Rhizoma Cimicifugae), *Bai Zhi* (Radix Angelicae Dahuricae), *Ge Gen* (Radix Puerariae), and *Gan Cao* (Radix Glycyrrhizae).

In case of thirst and a dry throat, turn to *Gan Ge* (dry Radix Puerariae) and *Hua Fen* (Radix Trichosanthis Kirlowii). For phlegm, *Bei Mu* (Bulbus Fritillariae) is considered best of all. For coughing, it is alright to add *Wu Wei Zi* (Fructus Schisandrae Chinensis) and *Sang Pi* (Cortex Radicis Mori Albi). For insomnia, it is appropriate to add *Suan Zao Ren* (Semen Zizyphi Spinosae). For food damage and low food intake, add *Shen Qu* (Massa Medica Fermentata), *Mai Ya* (Fructus Germinatus Hordei Vulgaris), *Zhi Shi* (Fructus Immaturus Citri Aurantii), and stir-fried *Shan Zha* (Fructus Crataegi). For upflaming vacuity fire, add *Zhi Mu* (Rhizoma Anemarrhenae Asphodeloidis) and *Huang Bai* (Cortex Phellodendri), and it will be still better to take them with *Xuan Shen* (Radix Scrophulariae Ningpoensis).

For internal heat, employ *Huang Qin* (Radix Scutellariae Baicalensis), *Huang Lian* (Rhizoma Coptidis Chinensis), and *Hua Fen* (Radix Trichosanthis Kirlowii).

Lack of strength in the lower body requires (addition of) *Du Zhong* (Cortex Eucommiae Ulmoidis) and *Niu Xi* (Radix Achyranthis Bidentatae). For weakness of the feet, add *Mu Gua* (Fructus Chaenomlis Lagenariae) and *Fang Ji* (Radix Stephaniae Tetrandrae). For generalized fever, *Di Huang* (Radix Rehmanniae) should be used uncooked.

For fright palpitations and fearful throbbing, decoct and take together with *Yuan Zhi* (Radix Polygalae Tenuifoliae), *Fu Shen* (Sclerotium Pararadicis Poriae Cocos), *Chang Pu* (Rhizoma Acori Graminei), and *Bai*

*Zi Ren* (Semen Biotae Orientalis). (Besides,) employ *Mai Dong* (Tuber Ophiopogonis Japonici), *Wu Wei Zi* (Fructus Schisandrae Chinensis), *Suan Zao* (Semen Zizyphi Spinosae), *Shan Yao* (Radix Paeoniae Lactiflorae), and *Shan Yu* (Fructus Corni Officinalis) in any case.

If *Liu Jun* (Six Gentlemen [Decoction]) is supplemented by *Yuan Zhi* (Radix Polygalae Tenuifoliae), *Yi Mi* (Semen Coicis Lachryma-jobi), *Dang Gui* (Radix Angelicae Sinensis), *Lian Rou* (Semen Nelumbinis Nuciferae), *Shan Zha* (Fructus Crataegi), *Shan Yao* (Radix Paeoniae Lactiflorae), *Jie Geng* (Radix Platycodi Grandiflori), *Huang Lian* (Rhizoma Coptidis Chinensis), *Bian Dou* (Semen Dolichoris Lablab), *Huang Qi* (Radix Astragali Membranacei), and *Shen Qu* (Massa Medica Fermentata), it will be able to invigorate and fortify original yang and assist the spleen and stomach. In case of yin vacuity taxation coughing, decoct these with *Ren Shen* (Radix Panacis Ginseng) subtracted. If urination is normal, *Bai Fu Ling* (Sclerotium Poriae Cocos) becomes superfluous. This prescription is appropriate in case of aversion to food and is miraculously efficacious for internal damage due to taxation and toil. The spleen is the root of later heaven and mother of the tens of thousands (of living) things. (Therefore,) additions and subtractions from the formula (*i.e.,* Four Gentlemen Decoction) should be made to benefit the spleen.

# Chapter Ten
# Song on Additions & Subtractions to *Si Wu Tang* (Four Materials Decoction)

*Si Wu* (Four Materials [Decoction]) is composed of *Chuan Xiong* (Radix Ligustici Wallichii), *Dang Gui* (Radix Angelicae Sinensis), *Bai Shao* (Radix Albus Paeoniae Lactiflorae), and *Di Huang* (Radix Rehmanniae). It is the best formula for various pathoconditions in women because it is able to regulate the menses, nourish the blood, and cure vacuity detriment. For troubles related to pregnancy and childbirth, no other formulas are better than it.

If *Ren Shen* (Radix Panacis Ginseng), *Bai Zhu* (Rhizoma Atractylodis Macrocephalae), *Fu Ling* (Sclerotium Poriae Cocos), and *Gan Cao* (Radix Glycyrrhizae) are added, this is called *Ba Zhen* (Eight Pearls [Decoction]). It is rapidly effective for qi vacuity and blood weakness.

*Shi Quan* (Ten [Ingredients] Completely [& Greatly Supplementing Decoction]) is a formula including *Rou Gui* (Cortex Cinnamomi Cassiae) and *Huang Qi* (Radix Astragali Membranacei) in addition. It greatly supplements the true origin and blood vacuity.

For weakness, one must add *Shen Su* (Ginseng & Perilla [Drink]),[1] and then this is called *Bu Xin* (Supplement the Heart [Decoction]). It is appropriate to administer if there is heart vacuity with scanty blood and

---

[1] *Shen Su Yin* (Ginseng & Perilla Drink) is composed of *Ren Shen* (Radix Panacis Ginseng), *Zi Su* (Folium Perillae Frutescentis), *Ge Gen* (Radix Puerariae), *Qian Hu* (Radix Peucedani), *Ban Xia* (Rhizoma Pinelliae Ternatae), *Chi Fu Ling* (Sclerotium Rubrum Poriae Cocos), *Bai Fu Ling* (Sclerotium Poriae Cocos), *Zhi Ke* (Fructus Citri Aurantii), *Jie Geng* (Radix Platycodi Grandiflori), *Chen Pi* (Pericarpium Citri Reticulatae), and *Gan Cao* (Radix Glycyrrhizae).

fright with dreams or postpartum contraction of cold. One need not make any [other] additions or subtractions. This prescription will bring miraculous effect.

Fever arising in the late afternoon is due to yin vacuity. If *Zhi Mu* (Rhizoma Anemarrhenae Asphodeloidis) and *Huang Bai* (Cortex Phellodendri) are added to the formula, this will be eliminated completely.

Steaming bone taxation fever requires (adding) *Chai Hu* (Radix Bupleuri), *Huang Qi* (Radix Astragali Membranacei), *Bie Jia* (Carapax Amydae Sinensis), and *Zhi Mu* (Rhizoma Anemarrhenae Asphodeloidis). This also necessitates *Di Gu Pi* (Cortex Radicis Lycii Chinensis).

If a woman suffers from a malaria-like disease during menstruation, this can be treated by combining the primary decoction with *Xiao Chai* (Minor Bupleurum [Decoction]).[2]

If the menses come during pregnancy from time to time, add *E Jiao* (Gelatinum Corii Asini) and *Ai Ye* (Folium Artemisiae Argyii) to stop fetal leaking.

(To treat) delayed menstruation due to shortness of blood, double the amount of *Shu Di* (cooked Radix Rehmanniae) and add wine-processed *Huang Qin* (Radix Scutellariae Baicalensis). Premenstrual pain is caused by qi blocking the channels (or menses). *Xiang Fu* (Rhizoma Cyperi Rotundi), *E Zhu* (Rhizoma Curcumae Zedoariae), and *San Leng* (Rhizoma Sparganii) can free the flow of the channels or menses.

For purplish black menses or menstruation ahead of schedule, add *Huang Qin* (Radix Scutellariae Baicalensis) and *Huang Lian* (Rhizoma Coptidis Chinensis) to the formula and *Dan Pi* (Cortex Radicis Moutan) as well.

---

[2]  See chapter 12 below.

If, due to subjection to cold and static menses, there is lower abdominal pain, do not hesitate to add *Tao Ren* (Semen Pruni Persicae), *Wu Yao* (Radix Linderae Strychnifoliae), and *Xiang Fu* (Rhizoma Cyperi Rotundi).

To treat blood desiccation menstrual block in thin persons, add *Tao Ren* (Semen Pruni Persicae) to the primary formula.

A pale colored (menstrual flow) in fat persons is ascribed to phlegm stasis. This requires combining *Er Chen* (Two Aged [Ingredients Decoction])[3] (and *Si Wu Tang*) into one.

(To treat) excessive menstrual flow, *Chai Hu* (Radix Bupleuri), *Huang Qin* (Radix Scutellariae Baicalensis), *Huang Lian* (Rhizoma Coptidis Chinensis), and *Huang Bai* (Cortex Phellodendri) can be added together. In addition, *Jing Jie* (Herba Schizonepetae Tenuifoliae), *Sheng Ma* (Rhizoma Cimicifugae), *Qiang Huo* (Radix Et Rhizoma Notopterygii) [stir-fried till black], and *Du Huo* (Radix Angelicae Pubescentis) should be added. When the qi is lifted, this will automatically be quieted and harmonized.

This formula plus *Ren Shen* (Radix Panacis Ginseng) and *Bai Zhu* (Rhizoma Atractylodis Macrocephalae) are able to quiet the fetus.

In case of abdominal pain during pregnancy, add *Sha Ren* (Fructus Amomi) and *Zi Su* (Folium Perillae Frutescentis), and then depression will be opened automatically.

An unusually enlarged abdomen is the disease of fetal water. (This is due to) heart and chest qi counterflow which may become as hard as a drum. This responds well to *Li Yu Tang* (Carp Decoction)[4] boiled with *Bai Zhu* (Rhizoma Atractylodis Macrocephalae) and *Fu Ling* (Sclerotium Poriae Cocos), subtracting *Di Huang* (Radix Rehmanniae) and *Chuan Xiong*

---

3  See chapter 11 below.

4  *Li Yu Tang* (Carp Decoction) is composed of *Li Yu* (Carp), *Bai Zhu* (Rhizoma Atractylodis Macrocephalae), *Fu Ling* (Sclerotium Poriae Cocos), *Dang Gui* (Radix Angelicae Sinensis), *Shao Yao* (Radix Paeoniae Lactiflorae), *Ju Hong* (Exocarpium Citri Erythrocarpae) and *Sheng Jiang* (uncooked Rhizoma Zingiberis).

(Radix Ligustici Wallichii) but adding *Jiang* (Rhizoma Zingiberis) and *Ju Pi* (Pericarpium Citri Reticulatae) to (*Si Wu Tang*).

If the fetal qi is disquieted with distention of the chest and diaphragm, (adding) *Zhi Ke* (Fructus Citri Aurantii), *Sha Ren* (Fructus Amomi) and *Zi Su* (Folium Perillae Frutescentis) may bring immediate relief.

Heart vexation in pregnant women is called fetal vexation. The best policy (of treating it) is to add *Fu Pi* (Pericarpium Arecae Catechu), *Gan Cao* (Radix Glycyrrhizae), *Zhi Zi* (Fructus Gardeniae Jasminoidis), and *Huang Bai* (Cortex Phellodendri).

The two flavors, *Chuan Xiong* (Radix Ligustici Wallichii) and *Dang Gui* (Radix Angelicae Sinensis), comprise *Fo Shou San* (Buddha's Hand Powder). Taking it towards childbirth safeguards a (smooth) delivery. If difficult delivery occurs, *Cao Shuang* (Pulvis Fumi Carbonisati) and *Bai Zhi* (Radix Angelicae Dahuricae) may go along with it.

*Jiang Tan* (carbonized Rhizoma Zingiberis) is good for postpartum fever. Because it is acrid and sweet, it is able to greatly supplement heart blood.

In case of profuse sweating, subtract *Chuan Xiong* (Radix Ligustici Wallichii) from the formula, and then take it without delay together with *Ren Shen* (Radix Panacis Ginseng), *Huang Qi* (Radix Astragali Membranacei), and *Fang Feng* (Radix Ledebouriellae Divaricatae).

Postpartum blood confusion may develop into blood dizziness with profuse lochia and fatigued essence spirit. A formula called *Qing Hun San* (Clear the Ethereal Soul Powder) can settle this blood dizziness. It is composed of *Ze Lan* (Herba Lycopi Lucidi), *Chuan Xiong* (Radix Ligustici Wallichii), *Ren Shen* (Radix Panacis Ginseng), *Dang Gui* (Radix Angelicae Sinensis), *Jing Jie* (Herba Schizonepetae Tenuifoliae), and *Gan Cao* (Radix Glycyrrhizae).

*Hei Shen* (Black Spirit [Powder]) is (*Si Wu Tang*) minus *Chuan Xiong* (Radix Ligustici Wallichii) but plus *Guan Gui* (tubiform Cortex Cinnamomi Cassiae), *Hei Jiang* (blackened Rhizoma Zingiberis), mix-fried *Gan Cao*

(Radix Glycyrrhizae), stir-fried *Hei Dou* (Semen Glycinis Hispidae), and uncooked *Pu Huang* (Pollen Typhae). It can clear the lochia, precipitate the placenta, and relieve abdominal pain. It is extraordinarily (more) efficacious if it is decocted with wine and brewed in child's urine.

Suppose there is a scanty lochia, but otherwise there is no disease and the essence spirit is good. If suddenly cold and heat with abdominal pain occur, then it is a wise choice to prescribe *Hei Shen San* (Black Spirit Powder).

Postpartum, it is necessary to take *Si Wu Tang* (Four Materials Decoction). In primiparas, it is always necessary to use *Jiao Jiang* (scorched Rhizoma Zingiberis). Using *Bai Shao* (Radix Albus Paeoniae Lactiflorae) postpartum may damage the life qi. A slimy diaphragm[5] is incompatible with *Shu Di* (cooked Radix Rehmanniae). Intestinal efflux[6] prohibits either *Di Huang* (Radix Rehmanniae) or *Dang Gui* (Radix Angelicae Sinensis). If sweating is profuse, *Chuan Xiong* (Radix Ligustici Wallichii) should be removed. For blood vacuity abdominal pain, *Bai Shao* (Radix Albus Paeoniae Lactiflorae) should be retained.[7] There are many secrets treasured within the additions and subtractions of *Si Wu Tang*.[8]

---

[5] This refers to no desire for food with a feeling of stuffiness around the diaphragm.

[6] Intestinal efflux means frequent bowel movements or diarrhea.

[7] This sentence is an exception to the general rule of not using *Bai Shao* (Radix Albus Paeoniae Lactiflorae) postpartum. If there is blood vacuity abdominal pain, its use is warranted.

[8] This sentence means that there is a lot for students to learn about modifying this formula.

# Chapter Eleven
# Song on Additions & Subtractions to *Er Chen Tang* (Two Aged [Ingredients] Decoction)

*E*r Chen (Two Aged [Ingredients Decoction]) is composed of *Ju Pi* (Pericarpium Citri Reticulatae), *Ban Xia* (Rhizoma Pinelliae Ternatae), *Fu Ling* (Sclerotium Poriae Cocos), and *Gan Cao* (Radix Glycyrrhizae). It cannot be treasured too dearly (as a formula to) clear the qi and transform phlegm. For narrowing above the diaphragm[1], add *Zhi Shi* (Fructus Immaturus Citri Aurantii) and *Jie Geng* (Radix Platycodi Grandiflori). When there is effulgent fire generating phlegm, it is better (to add) *Huang Qin* (Radix Scutellariae Baicalensis) and *Huang Lian* (Rhizoma Coptidis Chinensis).

If *Ren Shen* (Radix Panacis Ginseng) and *Bai Zhu* (Rhizoma Atractylodis Macrocephalae) are added, this formula is called *Liu Jun Tang* (Six Gentlemen Decoction). No other formula is better than this for fortifying the spleen and harmonizing the stomach. When there is cold phlegm in the middle stomach duct, to eliminate it, remove *Ren Shen* (Radix Panacis Ginseng) but add stir-fried *Xiang Fu* (Rhizoma Cyperi Rotundi) and *Sha Ren* (Fructus Amomi).

When overeating results in not being able to disperse food, add *Mai Ya* (Fructus Germinatus Hordei Vulgaris), *Shen Qu* (Massa Medica Fermentata), *Shan Zha* (Fructus Crataegi), and *Hou Po* (Cortex Magnoliae Officinalis) to regulate (the stomach). If *Zhi Shi* (Fructus Immaturus Citri Aurantii) and stir-fried *Huang Qin* (Radix Scutellariae Baicalensis) are also

---

[1]　This means chest oppression or distention.

35

added, then there will be no longer any worry if one has a vacuous body with a weak spleen and stomach.

Coughing with engenderment of phlegm is divided into cold and heat. If there is heat, add *Huang Qin* (Radix Scutellariae Baicalensis) and *Huang Lian* (Rhizoma Coptidis Chinensis) as well as *Zhi Ke* (Fructus Citri Aurantii) and *Jie Geng* (Radix Platycodi Grandiflori). For cold phlegm, combine *Zhi Ke* (Fructus Citri Aurantii) and *Sha Ren* (Fructus Amomi) with the original formula. When this (prescription) has transformed the qi, the phlegm in the chest will vanish on its own.

There is nothing serious about coughing due to external contraction of wind cold. It (can be cured by) *Er Chen* (Two Aged [Ingredients Decoction]) plus *Zhi Ke* (Fructus Citri Aurantii), *Jie Geng* (Radix Platycodi Grandiflori), *Qian Hu* (Radix Peucedani), *Zi Su* (Folium Perillae Frutescentis), *Ge Gen* (Radix Puerariae), *Xing Ren* (Semen Pruni Armeniacae), and *Sang Pi* (Cortex Radicis Mori Albi) which are able to clear the lungs and *Mu Xiang* (Radix Auklandiae Lappae) which regulates the qi. This is the formula called *Shen Su Yin* (Ginseng & Perilla Beverage).

*Er Chen* (Two Aged [Ingredients Decoction]) contains *Ban Xia* (Rhizoma Pinelliae Ternatae) whose nature is dry. In the case of blood vacuity or thirst, it is, (therefore,) unwanted. It should be replaced by *Bei Mu* (Bulbus Fritillariae) which has the specific effect of ridding (of phlegm). This then becomes a four materials decoction.

There are diseases engendered by wind phlegm. (These require adding) *Tian Ma* (Rhizoma Gastrodiae Elatae), *Bai Fu Zi* (Rhizoma Typhonii Gigantei), *Zao Jiao* (Fructus Gleditschiae Chinensis), and *Nan Xing* (Rhizoma Arisaematis).

Damp phlegm in the stomach may make the body flaccid. (To treat this,) combine *Bai Zhu* (Rhizoma Atractylodis Macrocephalae) and *Cang Zhu* (Rhizoma Atractylodis) with *Er Chen* (Two Aged [Ingredients Decoction]).

Fire depression in the chest may produce old (*i.e.*, recalcitrant) bound phlegm which is held up in the throat and cannot be exhausted by hacking. (To treat this,) one may add *Gua Lou* (Fructus Trichosanthis Kirlowii), *Xiang Fu* (Rhizoma Cyperi Rotundi), *Jie Geng* (Radix Platycodi Grandiflori), *Huang Lian* (Rhizoma Coptidis Chinensis), and *Zhi Ke* (Fructus Citri Aurantii), and a little *Yuan Ming Fen* (Mirabilitum Depuratum) as an assistant. Then phlegm will vanish on its own.

If phlegm lodges in the channels and limbs[2], add *Jiang Zhi* (Succus Rhizomatis Zingiberis) and *Zhu Li* (Succus Bambusae). If phlegm lodges in the rib-side[3], it may be eliminated by (adding) *Bai Jie Zi* (Semen Sinapis Albae). Phlegm in the spleen and stomach[4] requires *Zhi Shi* (Fructus Immaturus Citri Aurantii).

*Wen Dan Tang* (Warm the Gallbladder Decoction) is (*Er Chen Tang*) plus *Zhu Ru* (Caulis Bambusae In Taeniis) and *Zhi Shi* (Fructus Immaturus Citri Aurantii). It is the first (choice) for quieting the spirit and sweeping away phlegm.

If *Zhi Shi* (Fructus Immaturus Citri Aurantii) and *Nan Xing* (Rhizoma Arisaematis) are added, then this formula becomes *Dao Tan Tang* (Abduct Phlegm Decoction). This is able to disinhibit the diaphragm.

If *Gan Cao* (Radix Glycyrrhizae) and *Chen Pi* (Pericarpium Citri Reticulatae) are subtracted but *Zi Su* (Folium Perillae Frutescentis), *Hou Po* (Cortex Magnoliae Officinalis), *Da Zao* (Fructus Zizyphi Jujubae), and *Sheng Jiang* (uncooked Rhizoma Zingiberis) are added, the formula becomes *Qi Qi Tang* (Seven Qi Decoction). This dissipates depression, disperses phlegm, and rectifies the qi. It is (also) good when used to treat malign obstruction during pregnancy (*i.e.*, morning sickness).

---

[2] When phlegm pours into the channels and limbs, various troubles may arise, such as migratory pain in the limbs, chest fullness, pain in the shoulder and upper back, and reduced food intake. The pulse is usually slippery but arrhythmic.

[3] This problem is characterized by a gurgling sound or feeling on the side of the chest.

[4] Phlegm in the spleen and stomach may give rise to clamoring stomach, nausea, vomiting and retching, glomus, and so on.

Retching of blood is without exception due to intense stomach fire. If the retching is continual with a surging, rapid pulse, one should use without delay *Er Chen* (Two Aged [Ingredients Decoction]) plus *Zhi Shi* (Fructus Immaturus Citri Aurantii), *Zhu Ru* (Caulis Bambusae In Taeniis), and ginger-juice fried *Huang Lian* (Rhizoma Coptidis Chinensis). If (the sick person) has difficulty swallowing these medicinals, decoct them together with a little *Bing Lang* (Semen Arecae Catechu) and *Mu Xiang* (Radix Auklandiae Lappae). If the retching has continued for five or six days on end with distention and oppression in the heart which are exacerbated by pressure, add large amounts of *Zhi Shi* (Fructus Immaturus Citri Aurantii), *Hou Po* (Cortex Magnoliae Officinalis), *Huang Qin* (Radix Scutellariae Baicalensis), *Huang Lian* (Rhizoma Coptidis Chinensis), and *Bai Shao* (Radix Albus Paeoniae Lactiflorae). If there is (also) constipation, put in *Mang Xiao* (Mirabilitum) and *Da Huang* (Radix Et Rhizoma Rhei) and then it will be cured along with (the retching).

Clamoring stomach and eructation can be treated the same. They are both due to accumulated heat and collecting phlegm in the chest. They are not difficult to treat at all if one modifies *Er Chen* (Two Aged [Ingredients Decoction]) by adding *Shi Gao* (Gypsum Fibrosum), *Xiang Fu* (Rhizoma Cyperi Rotundi), *Nan Xing* (Rhizoma Arisaematis), and *Huo Xiang* (Herba Agastachis Seu Pogostemi).

For oppression and distention with acid regurgitation and acid vomiting, add fried *Shan Yu* (Fructus Corni Officinalis) and *Huang Lian* (Rhizoma Coptidis Chinensis) to the original formula.

Water collecting below the heart is called rheum. (To treat this,) add *Zhi Shi* (Fructus Immaturus Citri Aurantii), *Fu Ling* (Sclerotium Poriae Cocos), and *Zhu Ling* (Sclerotium Polypori Umbellati) to disinhibit urination and defecation.

All the above are methods for adding to and subtracting from *Er Chen* (Two Aged [Ingredients Decoction]). One should not impart these to unworthy people.

# Chapter Twelve
# Song on Additions & Subtractions to *Xiao Chai Hu Tang* (Minor Bupleurum Decoction)

*C*hai Hu (Radix Bupleuri), *Ban Xia* (Rhizoma Pinelliae Ternatae), *Ren Shen* (Radix Panacis Ginseng), *Huang Qin* (Radix Scutellariae Baicalensis), and *Gan Cao* (Radix Glycyrrhizae) are as precious as gems for *shao yang* channel disease. They are good for alternating fever and chills in the late afternoon with retching and pain in the rib-side.

Disease of this channel (*i.e.,* the *shao yang*) may combined with the *yang ming,* (with symptoms of) thirst, vexation, frequent dry retching, pain in the eyes, dry nose, and insomnia. (For this, add) *Ge Gen* (Radix Puerariae), *Zhi Mu* (Rhizoma Anemarrhenae Asphodeloidis), *Bai Shao* (Radix Albus Paeoniae Lactiflorae), and (wine) stir-fried *Huang Qin* (Radix Scutellariae Baicalensis).

If there is glomus and fullness in the heart with effulgent heat, adding *Zhi Shi* (Fructus Immaturus Citri Aurantii) and *Jie Geng* (Radix Platycodi Grandiflori) is effective. If glomus and fullness refuse to be loosened, combine (this formula) with *Xiao Xian Xiong Tang* (Minor Falling Chest Decoction).[1] If there is scanty sweating, parched lips, dry mouth with thirst, and no end to drinking water, (add) *Huang Lian* (Rhizoma Coptidis Chinensis) and *Gan Ge* (dry Radix Puerariae). What to do if there is still no resolution? Add a pinchful of *Zhu Ru* (Caulis Bambusae In Taeniis) and *Shi Gao* (Gypsum Fibrosum) each.

---

[1] See #3, chapter 14 below.

If, following perspiration, there is vigorous fever all over the body with vexation, raving, and dry retching as well as groaning, decoct and administer (the original formula) together with *Huang Lian Jie Du Tang* (Coptis Resolve Toxin Decoction).[2] One dose and (the sick person) will be safe and sound immediately. If there is vexatious thirst, diarrhea, and increasing fever, combine the original formula with *Si Ling* (Four [Ingredients] Poria [Powder]).[3]

If yellowing (*i.e.*, jaundice) with reddish urine arises, increase the amount of *Huang Qin* (Radix Scutellariae Baicalensis) and add *Huang Lian* (Rhizoma Coptidis Chinensis), *Zhi Mu* (Rhizoma Anemarrhenae Asphodeloidis), and *Huang Bai* (Cortex Phellodendri).

Hard stools and dry mouth with thirst require (adding) *Huang Lian* (Rhizoma Coptidis Chinensis), *Hou Po* (Cortex Magnoliae Officinalis), *Gua Lou* (Fructus Trichosanthis Kirlowii), and *Zhi Ke* (Fructus Citri Aurantii). If the stools remain hard, nonetheless, with fecal block, it is never a mistake to use *Da Chai Hu Tang* (Major Bupleurum Decoction).[4]

For generalized fever, aversion to wind, and no dry mouth, it is necessary to combine the original formula with *Gui Zhi Tang* (Cinnamon Twig Decoction).[5] If there are parched lips with intense vexatious thirst, put *Shi Gao* (Gypsum Fibrosum) and *Zhi Mu* (Rhizoma Anemarrhenae Asphodeloidis) in the original formula. If there is vexation in the chest with no retching, subtract *Ban Xia* (Rhizoma Pinelliae Ternatae) and *Ren Shen* (Radix Panacis Ginseng) from the original formula and add a large amount of *Gua Lou Ren* (Semen Trichosanthis Kirlowii).

---

[2] See #3, chapter 14 below.

[3] This formula is composed of *Zhu Ling* (Sclerotium Polypori Umbellati), *Fu Ling* (Sclerotium Poriae Cocos), *Ze Xie* (Rhizoma Alismatis), and *Bai Zhu* (Rhizoma Atractylodis Macrocephalae).

[4] This formula is given in #3, chapter 14 below.

[5] This formula is given in #3, chapter 14 below.

In case of thirst, remove *Ban Xia* (Rhizoma Pinelliae Ternatae) and add *Zhi Mu* (Rhizoma Anemarrhenae Asphodeloidis) and *Hua Fen* (Radix Trichosanthis Kirlowii). In case of abdominal pain, add *Bai Shao* (Radix Albus Paeoniae Lactiflorae) and subtract *Huang Qin* (Radix Scutellariae Baicalensis). Heat in the rib-side with abdominal pain requires stir-fried *Huang Lian* (Rhizoma Coptidis Chinensis) and *Bai Shao* (Radix Albus Paeoniae Lactiflorae). In case of profuse phlegm, *Bei Mu* (Bulbus Fritillariae) and *Gua Lou* (Fructus Trichosanthis Kirlowii) are safeguards. Retching requires adding *Jiang Zhi* (Succus Rhizomatis Zingiberis), *Zhu Li* (Succus Bambusae), and *Chen Pi* (Pericarpium Citri Reticulatae). For coughing, it is appropriate to add *Wu Wei Zi* (Fructus Schisandrae Chinensis). For hardness and pain in the rib-side, add *Qing Pi* (Pericarpium Citri Reticulatae Viride) and *Mu Li* (Concha Ostreae). *Fu Ling* (Sclerotium Poriae Cocos) is a ruling (*i.e.*, main, ingredient) for difficult urination and palpitations below the heart. When there is glomus with distention and fullness in the chest and rib-side, use *Mu Li* (Concha Ostreae) and *Gan Jiang* (dry Rhizoma Zingiberis). This is a secret kept by scholars.

In case of chest fullness with coughing, removing *Ren Shen* (Radix Panacis Ginseng) and *Da Zao* (Fructus Zizyphi Jujubae) and adding *Wu Wei Zi* (Fructus Schisandrae Chinensis) and *Gan Jiang* (dry Rhizoma Zingiberis) is good.

In case of fluid vacuity with fever and massive drinking, add *Mai Dong* (Tuber Ophiopogonis Japonici) and *Wu Wei Zi* (Fructus Schisandrae Chinensis) and remove *Ren Shen* (Radix Panacis Ginseng).

In case of stomach vacuity with sloppy (*i.e.*, loose) stools, the two materials, *Shao Yao* (Radix Paeoniae Lactiflorae) and *Zhu Ling* (Sclerotium Polypori Umbellati), can render help.

For seminal emission due to insecurity (of the essence gate) and yin vacuity, add *Mu Li* (Concha Ostreae). It is even better to (also) add *Zhi Mu* (Rhizoma Anemarrhenae · Asphodeloidis) and *Huang Bai* (Cortex Phellodendri).

41

In case of tidal fever with absence of thirst and a desire to wear (thick) clothes, substitute *Gui Zhi* (Ramulus Cinnamomi Cassiae) for *Ren Shen* (Radix Panacis Ginseng).

In case of spring warmth with fever, cough, and thirst, it is appropriate to add *Wu Wei Zi* (Fructus Schisandrae Chinensis) and *Gua Lou* (Fructus Trichosanthis Kirlowii) and remove *Ban Xia* (Rhizoma Pinelliae Ternatae).

In case of warm disease with aversion to heat rather than cold, substitute *Fu Ling* (Sclerotium Poriae Cocos) for *Chai Hu* (Radix Bupleuri) and *Ren Shen* (Radix Panacis Ginseng) and add *Gui Zhi* (Ramulus Cinnamomi Cassiae), *Ge Gen* (Radix Puerariae), *Bai Shao* (Radix Albus Paeoniae Lactiflorae), *Sheng Ma* (Rhizoma Cimicifugae), and *Da Zao* (Fructus Zizyphi Jujubae). If there is sore throat, (the sick person) has to taste *Gan Cao* (Radix Glycyrrhizae) and *Jie Geng* (Radix Platycodi Grandiflori) in addition.

In case of channel passage delay[6] with fullness in the chest and rib-side, retching and tidal fever, put *Mang Xiao* (Mirabilitum) in *Chai Hu Tang* ([Minor] Bupleurum Decoction).

In case of warm malaria[7] with thirst, vexation, and aversion to heat, mix *Shi Gao* (Gypsum Fibrosum) and *Zhi MuTang* (Rhizoma Anemarrhenae Aspheloidis) with *Xiao Chai Hu Tang* (Minor Bupleurum Decoction).

If cold damage has endured for (many) days, this is called channel passage (delay). If there is neither an exterior nor interior pattern, this (decoction) can be prescribed. If evils are abundant with weak original qi, add large amounts of *Mai Dong* (Tuber Ophiopogonis Japonici), *Wu Wei Zi* (Fructus Schisandrae Chinensis), and *Ren Shen* (Radix Panacis Ginseng). If a relapse due to food and taxation occurs after recovery and there is a vigorous fever, heart palpitations, phlegm and hasty breathing, it is necessary to combine *Wen Dan Tang* (Warm the Gallbladder

---

[6] If cold damage remains unresolved on the 13th day, this is called channel passage delay.

[7] This refers to malaria with only fever or serious fever and only slight chills.

42

Decoction) with the original formula. Administer these without delay, and the (sick) person will recover before long.

Fever which is better by day but worse at night is known as evil heat entering the blood chamber. This allows (adding) *Mu Dan Pi* (Cortex Radicis Moutan), *Sheng Di* (uncooked Radix Rehmanniae), *Huang Bai* (Cortex Phellodendri), *Huang Lian* (Rhizoma Coptidis Chinensis), and *Zhi Zi* (Fructus Gardeniae Jasminoidis). Additionally prescribe *Zhi Mu* (Rhizoma Anemarrhenae Asphodeloidis) and *Dang Gui* (Radix Angelicae Sinensis). In case of exacerbation by day but relief at night, find *Zhi Mu* (Rhizoma Anemarrhenae Asphodeloidis), *Huang Lian* (Rhizoma Coptidis Chinensis), *Zhi Zi* (Fructus Gardeniae Jasminoidis), and *Di Gu Pi* (Cortex Radicis Lycii Chinensis) (and add these to the original formula).

Suppose there is tidal fever unabating either by day or by night, add *Si Wu* (Four Materials [Decoction]) to the formula together with *Zhi Zi* (Fructus Gardeniae Jasminoidis) and *Huang Lian* (Rhizoma Coptidis Chinensis).

In case of fluid desiccation urinary and fecal stoppage following perspiration, remove *Ban Xia* (Rhizoma Pinelliae Ternatae) but add *Sheng Di* (uncooked Radix Rehmanniae), *Huang Qin* (Radix Scutellariae Baicalensis), *Bai Zhu* (Rhizoma Atractylodis Macrocephalae), *Chen Pi* (Pericarpium Citri Reticulatae), *Dang Gui* (Radix Angelicae Sinensis), *Bai Shao* (Radix Albus Paeoniae Lactiflorae), and *Mai Dong* (Tuber Ophiopogonis Japonici). If severe dryness remains as before (nonetheless), one should take the bother of changing to another treatment (method).

Why should *Chai Hu* (Radix Bupleuri) and *Huang Qin* (Radix Scutellariae Baicalensis) stand side by side in the main formula? Because they are bitter in flavor, they are able to effuse and transform evil heat. *Ban Xia* (Rhizoma Pinelliae Ternatae) is an appropriate (medicinal) for stopping retching and eliminating phlegm since its nature is able to downbear the qi and its flavor is intensely acrid.

43

When the exterior is insufficient, sweet (medicinals) can moderate this. *Ren Shen* (Radix Panacis Ginseng) and *Gan Cao* (Radix Glycyrrhizae) are center-moderators, while *Jiang* (Rhizoma Zingiberis) and *Da Zao* (Fructus Zizyphi Jujubae) are necessary (medicinals) for harmonizing the constructive and defensive. For harmonizing and resolving, there is nothing better than to use this (formula).

## Chapter Thirteen
# Song on Additions & Subtractions to *Ping Wei San* (Calm the Stomach Powder)

(To compose) *Ping Wei* (Calm the Stomach [Powder]), find *Chen Pi* (Pericarpium Citri Reticulatae), *Cang Zhu* (Rhizoma Atractylodis), *Hou Po* (Cortex Magnoliae Officinalis), and *Gan Cao* (Radix Glycyrrhizae). Able to harmonize and balance, this is used to fortify the spleen and to dry dampness. It is always employed when there is a satiated (feeling) and oppression in the chest as in food damage and when there is clamoring stomach and acid regurgitation.

When dietary irregularities have damaged the spleen and stomach, *Xiang Fu* (Rhizoma Cyperi Rotundi), *Sha Ren* (Fructus Amomi), *Zhi Shi* (Fructus Immaturus Citri Aurantii), and *Mu Xiang* (Radix Auklandiae Lappae) can render help.

For food accumulation, use stir-fried *Mai Ya* (Fructus Germinatus Hordei Vulgaris) and *Shen Qu* (Massa Medica Fermentata). For meat accumulation, *Shan Zha* (Fructus Crataegi) and *Cao Guo* (Fructus Amomi Tsao-ko) are good. For fruit retention, it is proper to put in *Gan Jiang* (dry Rhizoma Zingiberis) and *Qing Pi* (Pericarpium Citri Reticulatae Viride). For wine damage, add *Huang Lian* (Rhizoma Coptidis Chinensis), *Ge Hua* (Flos Puerariae), and *Wu Mei* (Fructus Pruni Mume). In case of retching and vomiting, do not forget *Ding Xiang* (Flos Caryophylli), *Wu Mei* (Fructus Pruni Mume), *Huo Xiang* (Herba Agastachis Seu Pogostemi), and *Ban Xia* (Rhizoma Pinelliae Ternatae). When accumulated heat is collecting so as to cause fecal stoppage, precipitate it with *Bing Lang* (Semen Arecae Catechu), *Zhi Shi* (Fructus Immaturus Citri Aurantii), and *Da Huang* (Radix Et Rhizoma Rhei). If there is accumulated cold causing difficult dispersion and transformation (of food), prescribe *Gan Jiang* (dry Rhizoma Zingiberis), *Rou Gui* (Cortex Cinnamomi Cassiae), *E Zhu* (Rhizoma Curcumae Zedoariae), *San Leng* (Rhizoma Sparganii), and *Ba Dou* (Semen Crotonis Tiglii).

When damp heat steams, producing a sour taste in the mouth, decoct *Xiang Fu* (Rhizoma Cyperi Rotundi) and *Sha Ren* (Fructus Amomi) together with stir-fried *Huang Lian* (Rhizoma Coptidis Chinensis), *Wu Zhu Yu* (Fructus Evodiae Rutecarpae), *Zhi Zi* (Fructus Gardeniae Jasminoidis), and *Zhi Shi* (Fructus Immaturus Citri Aurantii).

Clamoring stomach requires adding *Chuan Xiong* (Radix Ligustici Wallichii) and *Bai Shao* (Radix Albus Paeoniae Lactiflorae).

In case of failure to acclimatize to a new environment, adding *Xiang Fu* (Rhizoma Cyperi Rotundi), *Sha Ren* (Fructus Amomi), *Huo Xiang* (Herba Agastachis Seu Pogostemi), and *Ban Xia* (Rhizoma Pinelliae Ternatae) is wonderfully effective.

For vomiting and diarrhea, it is good to add *Fu Ling* (Sclerotium Poriae Cocos) and *Bai Zhu* (Rhizoma Atractylodis Macrocephalae), but it is still more wonderful to further add stir-fried *Yi Ren* (Semen Coicis Lachryma-jobi), *Shan Yao* (Radix Paeoniae Lactiflorae), and *Wu Mei* (Fructus Pruni Mume).

(To treat) diarrhea with nontransformation of food, *Wu Ling San* (Poria Five [Ingredients Powder])[1] is really a priceless match to combine with (*Ping Wei San*).

---

[1] This formula is composed of *Fu Ling* (Sclerotium Poriae Cocos), *Zhu Ling* (Sclerotium Polypori Umbellati), *Bai Zhu* (Rhizoma Atractylodis Macrocephalae), *Ze Xie* (Rhizoma Alismatis), and *Gui Zhi* (Ramulus Cinnamomi Cassiae).

Food stagnation with constant satiety is due to spleen vacuity. (To treat it,) add *Yi Gong* (Special Achievement [Powder])²along with *Xiang Fu* (Rhizoma Cyperi Rotundi) and *Sha Ren* (Fructus Amomi).

What is the prescription for sudden turmoil of vomiting and diarrhea? Substitute *Bai Zhu* (Rhizoma Atractylodis Macrocephalae) for *Cang Zhu* (Rhizoma Atractylodis) and tack on *Er Chen* (Two Aged [Ingredients Decoction]). Decoct and take these together with *Fu Pi* (Pericarpium Arecae Catechu), *Zi Su* (Folium Perillae Frutescentis), *Huo Xiang* (Herba Agastachis Seu Pogostemi), *Bai Zhi* (Radix Angelicae Dahuricae), *Sheng Jiang* (uncooked Rhizoma Zingiberis) and *Da Zao* (Fructus Zizyphi Jujubae). In case of cramping, add *Mu Gua* (Fructus Chaenomelis Lagenariae) to help. In case of abdominal pain, it is appropriate to add *Bai Shao* (Radix Albus Paeoniae Lactiflorae) and *Mu Xiang* (Radix Auklandiae Lappae). In case of cold (abdominal) pain, add *Gan Jiang* (dry Rhizoma Zingiberis), and *Rou Gui* (Cortex Cinnamomi Cassiae). For glomus and fullness, *Qing Pi* (Pericarpium Citri Reticulatae Viride) and *Zhi Shi* (Fructus Immaturus Citri Aurantii) are good.

For dry sudden turmoil with no vomiting or diarrhea³, add *Xiang Fu* (Rhizoma Cyperi Rotundi), *Sha Ren* (Fructus Amomi), *Mu Xiang* (Radix Auklandiae Lappae), *Zhi Ke* (Fructus Citri Aurantii), *Rou Gui* (Cortex Cinnamomi Cassiae), *Huo Xiang* (Herba Agastachis Seu Pogostemi), *Gan Jiang* (dry Rhizoma Zingiberis), and *Zi Su* (Folium Perillae Frutescentis) to the original formula.

For hardness and pain in the abdomen, *Bing Lang* (Semen Arecae Catechu) and *Shan Zha* (Fructus Crataegi) are efficacious.

---

2   This powder is composed of *Ren Shen* (Radix Panacis Ginseng), *Fu Ling* (Sclerotium Poriae Cocos), *Bai Zhu* (Rhizoma Atractylodis Macrocephalae), *Chen Pi* (Pericarpium Citri Reticulatae), and *Gan Cao* (Radix Glycyrrhizae).

3   Dry sudden turmoil refers to gripping abdominal pain, a desire but inability to vomit, a desire but inability to defecate, vexation and agitation, and, in extreme cases, a green-blue facial complexion, cold limbs, and a hidden pulse.

In case of cold stomach retching and vomiting, put in *Ding Xiang* (Flos Caryophylli). It is even better to also use *Rou Gui* (Cortex Cinnamomi Cassiae) and *Gan Jiang* (dry Rhizoma Zingiberis).

In case of vacuity sweating with green-blue lips and cold of the four limbs, remove *Chen Pi* (Pericarpium Citri Reticulatae) and add *Fu Zi* (Radix Lateralis Praeparatus Aconiti Carmichaeli) and *Hui Xiang* (Fructus Foeniculi Vulgaris).

# Chapter Fourteen
# Prose & Verse on Disease Causes

The generation of the hundreds of diseases each has its causes. When such a cause prevails somewhere (in the body), it will display certain signs and symptoms. These signs and symptoms are the ends (or branches) of the disease, while the cause is its root. Therefore, the *Nei Jing* (*The Inner Classic*) says:

> If one knows the root and ends (*i.e.*, branches), ten thousand attempts, ten thousands successes. Ignorance of the root and ends only leads to reckless action.

The hundreds of diseases all arise out of the six qi. None of the various diseases can escape the four causes. In relation to cold damage pathoconditions, one must become familiar with the six channel shift. In regard to scourge epidemic diseases, one must first be clear about contraction and offence of the four qi. As to internal damage of the spleen and stomach, one should identify superabundance and insufficiency. As to external contraction of febrile disease, one should know summerheat from spring warmth.

Sudden wind stroke has four causes and is classified into three categories in terms of treatment. Breaking and damaging wind (*i.e.*, lockjaw) is divided into three categories, and its treatment is based on the division of three channels. Summerheat stroke has stirring and still varieties. Dampness affection is separated into internal and external. There are seven species of fire, while phlegm has 10 causes. Concerning the qi, there are nine problems, and depression has six names. Malaria is due to assailment of summerheat wind but may be complicated by phlegm and food. The causes of dysentery are dampness, heat, and (food) collecting and accumulation. Retching and vomiting are caused by counterflow of the stomach qi which refuses to descend, while diarrhea is due to damaged, unbalanced spleen qi. Sudden turmoil is a result of spleen cold and food damage. Glomus fullness develops from a fatigued spleen and accumulated dampness. Hiccup is due to abnormality of the stomach qi.

Cough is due to the lung qi which is not clear. Eructation is invariably impugned to phlegm (or) fire. Acid swallowing is the work of food stagnation with no exception. Center fullness drum distention is due to a vacuous spleen failing to move. Dysphagia occlusion and stomach reflux are due to congealed qi and food.

Rapid panting is classified into vacuity and repletion. Tetany is classified into yin and yang.

The five accumulations and six gatherings are all due to qi-congealed phlegm and blood. The five taxations and six extremes are all due to fire scorching the heavenly true.

Blood ejection (*i.e.*, hematemesis) comes from the bowel of the stomach. Nosebleeding roots in the lung channel. Blood in phlegm drool is ascribed to the spleen viscus, while hacking and spitting of blood is ascribed to the kidney channel. Gaping gums are produced by extreme heat of the *yang ming*, and tongue bleeding arises from the fire of the *shao yin*.

In regard to abdominal constriction, this is divided into phlegm and fire. Vexatious heat in the chest is classified into vacuity and repletion.

Fright palpitations are caused by confounding phlegm and fear. Forgetfulness is a product of shortage of blood due to anxiety and depression.

In terms of mania and withdrawal, this is divided into extreme heat of the heart and that of the liver. In connection with epilepsy, one should detect serious and slight phlegm fire.

In relation to turbid urine, one should differentiate the red from the white. Sweating may be named spontaneous or night.

The nine kinds of heart pain are located in the stomach duct. The seven categories of mounting (*i.e.*, *shan*) qi are diseases of the *jue yin*.

Rib-side pain differs in the two sides. Head wind is separated as the left and right.

Lumbago is due to kidney vacuity or wrenching and contusion. Abdominal pain is due to cold qi or food stagnation. The pathocondition of wilting is due to insufficiency and damp heat. The pathocondition of impediment is caused by overwhelming cold, dampness, and wind.

The four categories of seminal emission are all due to noninteraction of the heart and kidneys. The five species of jaundice are produced by fuming and steaming damp heat.

Dizziness never arises without phlegm, while wasting thirst never occurs without fire.

Insomnia is due to effulgent phlegm fire and shortage of blood. Profuse sleeping is due to fatigued spleen and stomach and clouded spirit.

Constipation is due to dried and bound blood and liquids, while urinary block is due to stagnated qi failing to move.

Hemorrhoidal disease and intestinal wind are caused by damp heat. Macular eruptions and addictive papules are produced by overwhelming wind heat.

Deafness is a result of kidney vacuity, while the cause of ocular disease is liver fire. Toothache is due to stomach heat and worm erosion. Throat impediment is caused by stirring fire engendering phlegm. Nasal congestion is a manifestation of inhibited lung qi. Mouth sores are a product of wandering spleen fire.

Menstrual irregularities in women are all ascribed to qi counterflow. Heart vexation and tidal fever in women arise from depression in most cases. The cause of vaginal discharge and sand strangury is damp heat.

Flooding and leaking of blood is due to detriment of the *chong* and *ren*. Concerning disquieted fetus, there are two treatment principles. Postpartum fever has seven causes.

This essay is (only) an outline of seventy-four categories of disease. To know these in full, read the discussions which follow. Studying formulary is like studying law, whereas prescribing medicinals resembles commanding troops. One should never design a (military) strategy impetuously, and what is treasured in learning is proficient and perfect knowledge.[1]

# 1. The Hundreds of Diseases All Arise Out of the Six Qi

The six qi are wind, heat, dampness, fire, dryness, and cold. The *Yuan Bing Shi (The Formulated Origins of Diseases)*[2] says,

> All sudden rigidity, propping pain[3], vessel tugging, abdominal urgency, and sinew contraction are ascribed to wind. The qi of the liver and gallbladder is foot *jue yin* wind wood.

The various diseases of panting, retching, acid regurgitation, fulminant pouring (*i.e.*, drastic diarrhea), lower body distress, twisted sinews (*i.e.*, muscle cramps), turbid urine, abdominal distention and enlargement like a drum, welling abscesses, flat abscesses, sores, tumor qi, nodulations, sudden turmoil of vomiting and diarrhea, visual distortion, depression, swelling and distention, nasal congestion, runny nose and nosebleed,

---

[1] The above section is the outline of this chapter, and below, each sentence becomes a subheading under which the statement is discussed more fully.

[2] This is the abbreviated title of the *Su Wen Xuan Ji Yuan Bing Shi (The Formulated Origins of Diseases Based on the Intricate Mechanisms of the Simple Questions)* written by Liu Wan-su (1120-1200 CE).

[3] This refers to cramps with pain.

blood spillage[4], blood discharging[5], strangury, constipation, generalized fever, aversion to cold, shivering, fright, confusion, sorrow and laughter (*i.e.*, emotional lability), delirious raving, and black external bleeding are all ascribed to heat. The qi of the true heart and small intestine is the sovereign fire of the *shao yin*.

All tetany, rigidity, accumulated rheum, glomus around the diaphragm, center fullness, sudden turmoil of vomiting and diarrhea, generalized heaviness, and swollen instep (soft) like mud which is pitted when pressed are ascribed to dampness. The qi of the spleen and stomach is the damp earth of the foot *tai yin*.

All fever, distorted vision with tugging, sudden loss of voice, clouding (of consciousness), agitation and restlessness, mania with eccentric behavior and abusive language, fright, swollen, sore, aching instep, qi counterflow penetrating upward, clenched jaw with shivering with the spirit seeming to have lost its containment, snorting, retching, sores, throat impediment, ringing in the ears and deafness, projectile vomiting of food which will not descend, lack of clarity of vision, fulminant downpour diarrhea, and twitching and tugging of the muscles, sudden disease, and sudden death are ascribed to fire. (This fire) is the heat of the hand *shao yang* ministerial fire and the qi of the pericardium and triple burner.

All rough (skin), desiccation, dried sinews, and skin cracking are ascribed to dryness. The qi of the lungs and large intestine is dry metal of the hand *yang ming*.

The various diseases of clear, chilly liquid exited from the upper and lower (orifices), concretions and conglomerations, bulging mounting (*i.e.*, *tui shan*), hard glomus, abdominal fullness, urgency and pain, clear food diarrhea, prolonged satiety, vomiting and diarrhea of foul, fishy substances, and reverse flow with difficult bending and stretching (of the

---

[4]   This refers to bleeding from the upper orifices, for example, from the ears, nose or eyes.

[5]   This refers to blood in urine and stools.

limbs) are all ascribed to cold. The qi of the kidneys and urinary bladder is cold water of the foot *tai yang*.

Wind is classified as wind cold and wind heat. In case of wind cold, one should dispel wind by effusing and dissipating. Then wind will certainly be resolved. In case of wind heat, one should dissipate heat depression, and then wind will certainly be calmed.

Heat is classified as vacuity heat, replete heat, and heat depression. For vacuity heat, supplement. For replete heat, discharge. For heat depression, dissipate.

Dampness is divided into cold dampness, wind dampness, damp heat, and damp qi. For cold dampness, (use) hot medicinals to dry it. Wind dampness can be overcome with windy medicinals.[6] For damp heat, (use) cold medicinals to clear and disinhibit it. For damp qi[7], (use) qi medicinals[8] to free it.

Cold is classified as internal cold, external cold, and vacuity cold. In case of internal cold, warming the center should take precedence. External cold requires first effusing the exterior. (To treat) vacuity cold, one should invigorate yang and simultaneously secure the root.

Dryness is divided into heat dryness, cold dryness, and wind dryness. For heat dryness, clear heat. For cold dryness, warm the channels. For wind dryness, dispel wind. (However,) one must make medicinals that nourish the blood and moisten dryness sovereigns.

---

[6] This refers to medicinals that can treat wind, like *Fang Feng* (Radix Ledebouriellae Divaricatae) and *Qiang Huo* (Radix Et Rhizoma Notopterygii).

[7] Damp qi is contracted when one falls asleep while wet with sweat or immediately after bathing. This dampness may assail the kidneys causing swollen external kidneys (*i.e.*, testicles), lumbago, and rigidity of the spine.

[8] Medicinals like *Bing Lang* (Semen Arecae) and *Mu Xiang* (Radix Auklandiae Lappae) that free the qi are called qi medicinals.

# 2. None of the Various Diseases Escape the Four Causes

The four causes are qi, blood, phlegm, and food. When Dan-xi[9] treated disease, he used *Si Jun [Zi] Tang* (Four Gentlemen Decoction) to treat the qi, *Si Wu Tang* (Four Materials Decoction) to treat the blood, *Er Chen Tang* (Two Aged [Ingredients] Decoction) to treat phlegm, and *Ping Wei San* (Calm the Stomach Powder) to treat food. In treatment, he mostly used these four formulas as rulers, and sometimes made use of the method of (opening) depression. Therefore, although (he) did not use vastly varied medicinals, (he) struck most diseases.

# 3. In Relation to Cold Damage, One Must Be Familiar with the Six Channel Shift

From Frost's Descent to the Spring Equinox[10], cold damage diseases may occur with the six channel shift. When (the disease) has gone through the six channels, it should automatically heal.[11] If one has read the *Su Wen* (*The Simple Questions*), (one knows) this is not empty speech.

In a dual contraction cold damage condition, two channels are involved in one day with both the exterior and interior diseased. (The sick person) may suffer from inability to take in water and recognize people and they may lose their life within six days. Therefore, it is said that, even though one takes no medicinals, cold damage may not give trouble starting from

---

[9] Dan-xi (Cinnabar Creek) is the honorific name of Zhu Zhen-heng (1281-1358 CE), the founder of the School of Enriching Yin. He believed that yang is usually superabundant, while yin is usually insufficient. Zhu Zhen-heng was one of the so-called Four Great Masters of the Jin-Yuan dynasties.

[10] These are the 17th and 4th of the 24 nodes of qi of the traditional Chinese calendar.

[11] Cold damage should stay in one channel for one day. Therefore, it should have traversed all the six channels in six days, and, hence, it should heal without treatment on the seventh day as long as there are no complications and no aberration from this progression.

the seventh day on. Within these seven days, (however,) it only needs one mistaken prescription (for cold damage) to become a bad (*i.e.*, hazardous) condition, and then it is too late to remedy. One should be careful about exuberant yang repelling yin[12] and exuberant yin repelling yang.[13] These require special study. If one is well informed about the exterior and interior and yin and yang, one will never fail to make a right choice among diaphoresis, warming, ejection, and precipitation.

## Rhymes on Prescriptions for the *Tai Yang* Channel Pattern

The *tai yang* channel pattern starts with aversion to cold and manifests as generalized fever, headache, and pain in the spine. When there is sweating, it is (called) wind damage[14], and the pulse is floating and moderate, while if there is no sweating, it is (called) cold damage, and the pulse is tight and bowstring. If there is no sweating, one may use *Ma Huang Tang* (Ephedra Decoction)[15] to promote perspiration. For copious sweating, it is appropriate to decoct *Gui Zhi* (Cinnamon Twig [Decoction]). The popular formula, *Xiang Su Yin* (Cyprus & Perilla Beverage), can be used with (certain) additions and subtractions when the (*tai yang*) channel is struck by disease. This will effect an instant cure. (Cold damage) disease begins with the *tai yang*, and immediate effusion of the exterior may effect recovery in no time. If medicinals for the *yang ming* are misused (to treat the *tai yang*), rather than cooling, heat will be drawn into the muscles.

---

[12] This is true heat in the interior with false cold in the exterior.

[13] This means that there is true cold in the interior while the exterior manifests heat, such as a red face, fever, and vexation.

[14] Wind damage is one type of cold damage. It is characterized by spontaneous sweating.

[15] This formula is composed of *Ma Huang* (Herba Ephedrae), *Gui Zhi* (Ramulus Cinnamomi Cassiae), *Gan Cao* (Radix Glycyrrhizae), and *Xing Ren* (Semen Pruni Armeniacae).

## Rhymes on Prescriptions for the *Yang Ming* Channel Pattern

The *yang ming* channel pattern manifests as fever (as high) as boiling water, no aversion to cold, (desire to) reduce one's clothes, pain in the eyes, dry nose, insomnia, and a floating, surging, slippery, rapid, and long pulse. Its (treatment) method is to resolve the muscles through slightly promoting perspiration. (To do this,) *Sheng Ma Ge Gen Tang* (Cimicifuga & Pueraria Decoction) is the best choice. When disease has shifted from the *tai yang* to the *yang ming*, the prescription of *Sheng Ma Ge Gen Tang* (Cimicifuga & Pueraria Decoction) may effect relief in no time. If *Xiao Chai Hu Tang* (Minor Bupleurum Decoction) is misused, the evil will shift into the *shao yang* channel.

## Rhymes on Prescriptions for the *Shao Yang* Channel Pattern

The *shao yang* (pattern) manifests as alternating fever and chills, dry mouth and throat, pain in the chest and rib-side, dry retching, a bowstring pulse, and impaired hearing. *Xiao Chai Hu* (Minor Bupleurum [Decoction]) may effect harmonization and resolution (of the exterior and interior) to bring about peace and quietude. When (disease) has shifted from the *yang ming* to the *shao yang* channel, one dose of *(Xiao) Chai Hu* (Minor Bupleurum Decoction) will clear heat immediately. If *Ma Huang (Tang)* (Ephedra [Decoction]) is used to double diaphoresis, (the pattern) will transform into blood amassment with steaming fever. Before the *shao yang* channel pattern is completely eradicated, if the General[16] is used to precipitate, it will give rise to vacuity, and hence glomus qi and chest binding. Please bear this in mind in treating disease.

## Rhymes on Prescriptions for the *Tai Yin* Channel Pattern

The *tai yin* channel pattern should manifest as aversion to heat, a deep, forceful pulse with no interruption, a tongue with fur, and rapid breathing in addition to vexation and agitation. (In that case,) do not be afraid of prescribing *Shi Gao Zhi Mu (Tang)* (Gypsum & Anemarrhena

---

[16] The General is another name of *Da Huang* (Radix Et Rhizoma Rhei). However, here it implies any drastically precipitating medicinals.

Decoction). If the *tai yin* (pattern) displays aversion to heat, vexation and agitation, a dry mouth, a tongue with fur, oppression below the heart, uninhibited urination and defecation, then the disease lies in the center. It will respond best to *Huang Lian Xie Xin Tang* (Coptis Drain the Heart Decoction). Since the *tai yin* (pattern) includes aversion to heat, thirst in most cases, vexation and agitation, abdominal fullness, and frequent bowel movements, it needs both *Huang Qin* (Radix Scutellariae Baicalensis) and *Huang Lian* (Rhizoma Coptidis Chinensis), and besides, *Gan Cao* (Radix Glycyrrhizae) as a center-harmonizer. If, in addition to aversion to heat, the *tai yin* channel pattern exhibits critical (signs like) abdominal pain and abdominal binding[17], *Gui Zhi Da Huang Tang* (Cinnamon Twig & Rhubarb Decoction) can bring a most rapid effect. If, in the *tai yin* channel pattern, there is still heat in the exterior with vexation, agitation, and bound stools in the interior, and if there are fullness and oppression in the abdomen and a tongue with fur, *Da Chai Hu Tang* (Major Bupleurum Decoction) can overcome this in no time.

## Rhymes on Prescriptions for the *Shao Yin* Channel Pattern

The *shao yin* channel pattern manifests as a cool body, aversion to heat, vexation and agitation, flailing of the arms and legs, thirst, tongue fur, fullness and hardness in the abdomen, and fecal and urinary stoppage with manic speech or diarrhea with purely clear water. All this is ascribed to evil heat hidden in the stomach. The (treatment) method is to use a bitter, cold formula of offensive precipitation, administering the three-flavor *Xiao Cheng Qi Tang* (Minor Order the Qi Decoction) without delay.

## Rhymes on Prescriptions for the *Jue Yin* Channel Pattern

The *jue yin* channel pattern manifests as generalized reversal cold, vexation and agitation, stripping of clothes, fullness and hardness of the abdomen, a curled tongue and retracted testicles, and upward surging of the qi. If mania with raving arises, life is in peril. The advice for the (attending) physician is not to scuttle (around not knowing what to do).

---

[17] Abdominal binding here means abdominal fullness and pain and constipation.

To know life and death, one can scrutinize the pulse. A pulse suggesting life comes deep and forceful. (In that case,) administer *Da Cheng Qi (Tang)* (Major Order the Qi Decoction) without delay, and then recovery will ensue. A pulse suggesting death comes faint and chaotic. (In that case,) it is futile to prescribe any formula.

Reverse flow in the three yin patterns are not true cold but false cold. In spite of reversal cold in the exterior, there is replete heat in the interior. The *Nei Jing (Inner Classic)* says, "Hyperactivity is always harmful, while balance is order." When heat goes to the extreme, it may contrarily be complicated by cold transformation. Exuberant yang repels yin. As the heat is profound, so the reversal (cold) is profound. Although there is reversal cold in the exterior, this cannot be compared to aversion to cold in the *tai yang* pattern.

If disease starts with the *tai yang* and later shifts to the three yin one by one, then, at first, there must be flailing of the arms and legs, removing the quilts and clothes, mania and restlessness, and urinary and fecal stoppage. Then (the disease) will further progress to tranquility and reverse flow (cold). At this moment, the (attending) physician should make a close observation of the pathocondition. If one misuses hot medicinals, it is near to killing the (sick) person.

## Rhymes on Prescriptions for the True Cold Pattern of Direct Strike to the Three Yin

When debilitated original qi renders it easy for evils to invade, cold evils may directly strike the three yin. To treat these patterns of the three yin channels, one should differentiate them and be careful not to be confused about them owing to lack of mindfulness.

In the event of direct strike on the *tai yin*, there is aversion to cold and the pulse is deep, slow, bowstring, slippery, and faint. There is abdominal pain with the complication of vomiting and diarrhea. (To treat this,) administer one cup of *Li Zhong* (Rectify the Center [Decoction]) without delay.

Direct strike on the *tai yin* may exhibit aversion to cold complicated by fever, endless diarrhea, headache, generalized pain, and abdominal pain. This requires *Gui Zhi* (Ramulus Cinnamomi Cassiae), *Ren Shen* (Radix Panacis Ginseng), stir-fried *Bai Zhu* (Rhizoma Atractylodis Macrocephalae), *Jiang* (Rhizoma Zingiberis), and *Gan Cao* (Radix Glycyrrhizae).

In the event of direct strike on the *tai yin*, if the pulse is deep and faint, there may be reversal flow (cold and) pain in the four limbs as if flogged, and a ghastly facial complexion with insufficient (*i.e.*, lack of) spirit. Urination and defecation may be uninhibited. The appropriate (formula for this condition) is *Si Ni* (Four Counterflows [Decoction]).

Direct strike on the *shao yin* may manifest as generalized aversion to cold, fever, headache, a somber facial complexion, (pain in) the body as if flailed, and absence of sweating. This requires *Ma Huang Fu Zi Xi Xin Tang* (Ephedra, Aconite & Asarum Decoction). This pattern is seemingly like the *tai yang* (pattern). Then why is it taken as *shao yin*? The pulse is deep, slow, and choppy. Therefore, one should prescribe a decoction for warming the channel and effusing the exterior.

If direct strike on the *shao yin* manifests as aversion to cold and wind, generalized fever, headache, severe generalized pain, no thirst, and sweating, this will yield to *Gui Zhi* (Ramulus Cinnamomi Cassiae), *Fu Zi* (Radix Lateralis Praeparatus Aconiti Carmichaeli), and *Gan Cao* (Radix Glycyrrhizae). Why is this pattern categorized as the *shao yin*? Because the pulse is deep and faint and there is profound aversion to cold. Although there is heat in the exterior, this heat is not true heat. One should bear in mind that this is exuberant yin repelling yang.

Direct strike on the *jue yin* may manifest as generalized reversal cold and lower abdominal pain radiating to the penis. The pulse is deep, slow, bowstring, and faint. The appropriate (formula for this) is *Dang Gui Si Ni Tang* (Dang Gui Four Counterflows Decoction).

The cold pattern of direct strike on the three yin may manifest aversion to cold, no generalized fever, a green-blue facial complexion, no thirst, uninhibited urination and defecation, and a deep, slow pulse. This is familiar to everyone. If (its manifestations) are unusual, it may, (however,) be really hard to identify. For example, there may be generalized fever, a red face, uninhibited urination and defecation, and dry mouth. When a doctor comes across this, they should make a study of the pulse. Suppose, although large, it is vacuous, gaping, and forceless and there is no thirst, or, though it is deep, slow, bowstring, slippery, and faint, there is an insufficiency in the physical form and qi. This is a cold pattern. This may also be the result of unabating generalized fever in spite of administration of cool medicinals. It is not true heat, but false heat. Because cold evils are too exuberant, they force vacuity fire outward, which then meanders in the exterior. The *Nei Jing (Inner Classic)* says, when exuberant yin repels yang, if one is not observant and makes up a bitter, cold prescription, it will undoubtedly cause death.

Generally speaking, in relation to cold damage pathoconditions, if the yang pattern displays a yin pulse, it will end in death, but a yin pattern displaying a yang pulse suggests life (*i.e.*, survival). The evils in cold damage are external evils. It is the original qi that can stand up against it. The original qi is ascribed to yang. Therefore, when a yang pulse appears, there is life. When a yin pulse appears, it portends death. This is because the original qi has expired. The yang pulse is a pulse which is large, forceful, and not chaotic. The yin pulse is a pulse which is small, vacuous, faint, and extremely chaotic.

To design a treatment scheme for cold damage, it is necessary first to identify the pattern. After one is clear about yin and yang, exterior and interior, cold and heat, vacuity and repletion, one should carefully weigh the treatment methods of diaphoresis, ejection, precipitation, warming, or harmonizing. Thus one will never go wrong.

It is necessary first to observe the two eyes to see whether they are red or yellow. Then observe the mouth and tongue and see if there is fur. And finally, palpate from the cardiac region and chest down to the lower abdomen to see if there is pain or fullness anywhere. Next, one should inquire (of the patient) about their bitterness (*i.e.*, suffering), predilections, diet, and way of life, asking whether their urination and defecation are inhibited or uninhibited, whether they have taken any medicinals, and whether they have been treated with diaphoresis or precipitation. One must be well informed on all of this and correlate the pulse and the pattern before one can be free from mistakes in prescription.

A. In examining cold damage, one should first observe the two eyes and see whether they are red or yellow. If they are red, there is yang toxins. If, (in addition,) the six pulses are surging, large, and forceful with distressing thirst, then prescribe *San Huang Shi Gao Tang* (Three Yellows & Gypsum Decoction) for a mild case but *Da Cheng Qi Tang* (Major Order the Qi Decoction) for a severe case.

B. Then examine the mouth and tongue and see if there is fur. If the tongue fur is white, evils have not yet entered the interior and (the pathocondition) is categorized as a midstage pattern. This requires *Xiao Chai Hu Tang* (Minor Bupleurum Decoction) for harmonization and resolution (of the exterior and interior). If the tongue fur is yellow, evil heat is shown to be in the bowel of the stomach. This requires *Tiao Wei Cheng Qi Tang* (Regulate the Stomach & Order Qi Decoction) to precipitate (this heat). Precipitation, (however,) is allowed only when the stools are dry and solid, the pulse is deep and forceful, and there is intense thirst. If black fur grows over a prickly tongue, this is kidney water restrained by heart fire. One should use *Da Cheng Qi Tang* (Major Order the Qi Decoction) to precipitate (fire) without delay for evil heat is very severe. If there is thick dry tongue fur in cold damage, one may soak a piece of black cloth in well water and wash the tongue with it. Then scrape (the tongue) with a fresh piece of ginger repeatedly. The fur will then disappear on its own.

C. Next, palpate the cardiac region and chest down to the lower abdomen to see if there is pain anywhere.

i. If there is hardness and pain below the heart which is exacerbated by pressure, distressing thirst, and raving, if the stools are solid, and if the pulse is deep, replete, and forceful, this is chest binding. Without delay, one should use *Da Xian Xiong Tang* (Major Falling Chest Decoction) plus *Zhi Ke* (Fructus Citri Aurantii) and *Jie Geng* (Radix Platycodi Grandiflori) to precipitate (this binding).

ii. If the sick person feels full and oppressed in the heart and chest but this produces no pain when pressed, this is glomus fullness. It requires *Xie Xin Tang* (Drain the Heart Decoction) plus *Zhi Ke* (Fructus Citri Aurantii) and *Jie Geng* (Radix Platycodi Grandiflori). (This prescription) is magically effective.

iii. If, on palpation, hardness and pain are found in the lower abdomen, one should ask if urination is inhibited. If urination is uninhibited but the stools are black, possibly complicated by generalized yellowing, raving, distressing thirst, and a deep, replete pulse, it is known that blood amassment lies in the lower burner. This requires *Tao Ren Cheng Qi Tang* (Persica Order the Qi Decoction). When black substances are precipitated out, recovery will follow.

iv. If palpation finds distention and fullness in the lower abdomen without hardness or pain and urination is inhibited, it is known that fluids are held up and bound, (*i.e.*, urination is difficult). This requires *Wu Ling San* (Five [Ingredients] Poria Powder) plus *Mu Tong* (Caulis Akebiae) and *Zhi Zi* (Fructus Gardeniae Jasminoidis) to disinhibit (urination). Disinhibition, however, should not be carried out in a big way for fear that fluids may be exhausted.

D. To treat (patients with) cold damage who suffer from vexatious thirst with desire for water—desire for external water to help when water is wasted and exhausted internally—only give them one bowl even if, in great thirst, they desire to drink one *sheng*. It is better to give them too little rather than too much water. If they drink a great amount of water to their heart's content, water will collect below the heart and result in chest binding. Should the water be ejected into the lungs, panting and coughing will develop. If the water is retained in the stomach, dysphagia and retching will arise. If the water spills into the skin, swelling will be produced. If it gathers in the lower burner, dribbling urinary block will arise. If it percolates into the intestines, diarrhea will arise. All this is impugned to excessive drinking. Do not refuse (the sick person) water, nor should water be imposed on them. It is proper to give them water frequently but in small amounts.

E. To treat cold damage (lasting) more than 10 days still with exterior symptoms indicating diaphoresis, one may prescribe *Qiang Huo Chong He Tang* (Notopterygium Harmonious Flow Decoction) to promote moderate sweating. If more than 10 day old cold damage (presents) interior symptoms indicating precipitation, one may use *Da Chai Hu Tang* (Major Bupleurum Decoction) for the purpose of precipitation. After cold damage has gone through the channel passage, the righteous qi is usually vacuous. (Now) *Ma Huang Tang* (Ephedra Decoction) and *Cheng Qi Tang* (Order the Qi Decoction) are probably too drastic. If *Ma Huang Tang* (Ephedra Decoction) is misused, this will cause yang collapse in the (sick) person. If *Cheng Qi Tang* (Order the Qi Decoction) is misused, this will cause incessant diarrhea in the (sick) person.

Suppose there is an exterior pattern yet to be eliminated while an interior pattern is urgent, then there is no other choice but to apply precipitation. However, one can only mete out a moderate treatment by using *Da Chai Hu Tang* (Major Bupleurum Decoction) to free the exterior and interior. Moreover, if old and weak people or people with vacuity of both qi and blood have a pattern indicating precipitation, one should also use *Da Chai Hu Tang* (Major Bupleurum Decoction) for the purpose of precipitation. This can avoid damaging their original qi. The case, however, is different with (people of) robust age and strong physique. They should be treated in accordance with their disease.

F. Suppose there is headache, fever, and aversion to cold at the onset. Later, (the disease) transmits into the interior. If, by now, headache and fever are relieved but instead aversion to heat, thirst, and raving; tidal fever, spontaneous sweating, and constipation; stripping of quilts and clothes and flailing of the arms and legs; or macular eruption, yellowing, mania and restlessness have arisen, this is a heat pattern transmitting from the yang channel, the exterior, into the yin channel. This requires interior-attacking medicinals for precipitation.

If precipitation is not carried out when it ought, a transmuted pattern may arise with the hands and feet sometimes cold and sometimes warm. This is reversal due to yang which has gone to extreme. It is a yang pattern resembling a yin and is called yang reversal. (However,) although there is reversal cold externally, there is heat evil, internally. This requires *Cheng Qi Tang* (Order the Qi Decoction) to precipitate (this heat).

There are also cases where failure to carry out diaphoresis and precipitation or prescription of hot medicinals for a yang pattern make heat toxins penetrate (more) deeper. (As a result,) yang qi is solitarily exuberant, while yin qi sustains utter expiry. (The sick person) runs about naked, climbing on high, singing, cursing, and shouting, deadly thirsty with a red face and eyes. There is macular eruption and generalized yellowing, possible pure clear water diarrhea, or diarrhea with yellow and reddish stools. The six pulses are surging and large. This is named yang toxins macular pattern. For a mild case, prescribe *Xiao Ban Qing Dai Yin* (Disperse Macules Indigo Beverage). For severe cases, use *San Huang Shi Gao Tang* (Three Yellows Gypsum Decoction) removing *Ma Huang* (Herba Ephedrae) and *Dou Chi* (Semen Praeparatus Sojae) and adding *Da Huang* (Radix Et Rhizoma Rhei) and *Mang Xiao* (Mirabilitum) for the purpose of precipitation. (This prescription) recovers yin qi and promotes massive perspiration. Then a resolution will ensue.

G. In the initial stage of disease, there may be no headache or generalized fever, but there is fear of cold, reversal cold of the four limbs, abdominal pain, vomiting and diarrhea, covering up with quilts with the body curling up, and no thirst. Or there is shivering, the face is haggard as if scraped by a knife, and drool foaming at the mouth. The pulse is deep, thin, and forceless. This is direct strike by cold evils to the yin channel, (*i.e.*, a true cold pattern). (The evils) do not come from the yang channel. This requires warming with hot medicinals. If cold has gone to extreme, causing reversal cold of the hands and feet to extend beyond the elbows and knees, this is reversal started by excessive cold. It is called yin reversal, requiring warming with *Si Ni Tang* (Four Counterflows Decoction).

H. The various cases of abdominal fullness and abdominal pain are a yin pattern. There is, however, a difference in severity or slightness, and it is hardly possible to treat them with the same method. Abdominal pain with constipation requires *Gui Zhi Jia Shao Yao Tang* (Cinnamon Twig Decoction Plus Peony). For severe abdominal pain, use *Gui Zhi Da Huang*

*Tang* (Cinnamon Twig & Rhubarb Decoction). For loose bowels with abdominal pain and clear urine, it is necessary to apply warming with *Li Zhong Tang* (Rectify the Center Decoction) and *Si Ni Tang* (Four Counterflows Decoction). One should prescribe in accordance with (the degree of) severity or slightness. For a mild case, use *Wu Ji San* (Five Accumulations Powder). For a severe case, use *Si Ni Tang* (Four Counterflows Decoction).

I. There is also external contraction of cold evils, which, at the very beginning, is accompanied by chilled, uncooked food damage internally. As there is yin hidden internally, there is cold both internally and externally. Another possible (cause of this condition) is administration of cool medicinals by mistake in a true yin (pattern). Because yin qi is solitarily exuberant while yang sustains utter expiry, once the disease starts, there is reversal cold of the hands and feet, rigidity and heaviness of the upper and lower back, headache, pain in the eye sockets, retching and vomiting, vexation, oppression, diarrhea, abdominal pain, and (pain) all over the body as if flogged. The six pulses are deep and fine, and there is thirst yet with no desire to drink. Later, the toxic qi gradually penetrates deeper, entering the abdomen and assaulting the heart. Then there is inhibited throat and abdominal pain becomes severe. Distention and fullness below the heart arise which is as hard as a stone. There is unbearably intense thirst, incessant cold sweating, and possible mussitation. The nails become blackish green-blue. This is called a yin toxins pattern. One should moxa without delay *Guan Yuan* (CV/4) and *Qi Hai* (CV/6) 20-30 cones or iron the umbilicus with (heated) scallion, and orally administer *Hui Yang Ji Jiu Tang* (Recover Yang Emergency Decoction). When yang qi is recovered and a massive perspiration is promoted, resolution will follow.

J. If, in cold damage, the sick person becomes so manic, running about, that people are unable to subdue them, it is appropriate to light a fire in the sick person's room and pour a big bowl of vinegar over the fire. Then make the sick person sniff (the resulting fumes) and they will become quiet.

K. If there is incessant nosebleeding in cold damage, one may stick a wet piece of paper to the forehead (of the sick person) and then blow into the nose powdered stir-fried *Zhi Zi* (Fructus Gardeniae Jasminoidis). Then the bleeding will be stanched. This method, however, can be used only for enduring incessant bleeding. If the nose bleeds merely in drops, evils are (but) in the channel, yet to be eliminated, and this method cannot be applied.

L. Both cold damage and summerheat damage manifest fever, and one must distinguish between them. Cold damages the physical form, and summerheat damages the qi. Cold damage displays aversion to cold and a tight pulse. Summerheat damage displays aversion to heat and a vacuous pulse. These are the differences between them.

M. Before entering the house of (a person suffering from) scourge epidemic, one should put some sesame oil into their nose. Then infection can be avoided. On leaving, one should probe the nostrils with a paper quill to provoke snorting. Another method is to mix sesame oil with powdered *Xiong Huang* (Realgar) and *Cang Zhu* (Rhizoma Atractylodis) and put the mixture into the nose or to mix powdered *Xiong Huang* (Realgar) with water and put this into the nose. This can protect one from infection even if one sleeps with the sick person in the same bed.

*Ma Huang Tang* (Ephedra Decoction)

*Ma Huang Tang* includes *Gui Zhi* (Ramulus Cinnamomi Cassiae), *Xing Ren* (Semen Pruni Armeniacae), and *Gan Cao* (Radix Glycyrrhizae).[18] It is used when cold damage patterns with no sweating require effusing the exterior without delay.

---

[18] To save space, in most cases the author leaves out the ingredient(s) explicitly indicated by the formula name. Sometimes the author seems to give no components but a formula name. In that case, all the ingredients are contained in the formula name. In addition, it is noticeable that, in some places, the author uses a shortened name instead of the full one in writing out its composition. This does not mean two different formulas.

*Gui Zhi Tang* (Cinnamon Twig Decoction)

*Gui Zhi Tang* includes *Shao Yao* (Radix Paeoniae Lactiflorae), *Da Zao* (Fructus Zizyphi Jujubae), *Jiang* (Rhizoma Zingiberis), and *Gan Cao* (Radix Glycyrrhizae). It is able to effuse and dissipate evils in the defensive to abate cold damage with sweating.

*Xiang Su Yin* (Cyperus & Perilla Drink)

*Xiang Su Yin* uses *Zi Su* (Folium Perillae Frutescentis) and *Xiang Fu* (Rhizoma Cyperi Rotundi) in large amounts. Besides, there are *Chen Pi* (Pericarpium Citri Reticulatae) and *Gan Cao* (Radix Glycyrrhizae). It harmonizes and pacifies both the exterior and interior.

*Ge Gen Tang* (Pueraria Decoction)

*Ge Gen Tang* includes *Shao Yao* (Radix Paeoniae Lactiflorae), *Gan Cao* (Radix Glycyrrhizae), *Gui Zhi* (Ramulus Cinnamomi Cassiae), and *Ma Huang* (Herba Ephedrae). It treats the combined (pattern of) *tai yang* and the *yang ming* with absence of sweating requiring diaphoresis.

*Sheng Ma Ge Gen Tang* (Cimicifuga & Pueraria Decoction)

In *Sheng Ma Ge Gen Tang*, *Shao Yao* (Radix Paeoniae Lactiflorae) and *Gan Cao* (Radix Glycyrrhizae) help one another. One dosage is enough to effect recovery from the *yang ming* (pattern) with generalized fever.

*Shi Gao Zhi Mu Tang* (Gypsum & Anemarrhena Decoction)

*Shi Gao* (Gypsum Fibrosum) plus *Zhi Mu* (Rhizoma Anemarrhenae Asphodeloidis) are decocted together with *Gan Cao* (Radix Glycyrrhizae) and *Jing Mi* (Semen Oryzae Sativae). This (formula) is called for when there is vexatious thirst and rapid breathing and the pulse is replete.

*Huang Lian Xie Xin Tang* (Coptis Drain the Heart Decoction)

*Huang Lian Xie Xin Tang* is composed of one flavor. Five *qian* is decocted per dose together with 20 pieces of *Deng Xin* (Medulla Junci Effusi).[19] It calms and quiets vexation and fever in no time.

*Huang Qin Tang* (Scutellaria Decoction)

*Huang Qin Tang* includes *Shao Yao* (Radix Paeoniae Lactiflorae) and *Gan Cao* (Radix Glycyrrhizae) together with *Da Zao* (Fructus Zizyphi Jujubae), 2 pieces. Taking it warm is magically efficacious.

*Gui Zhi Jia Da Huang Tang* (Cinnamon Twig Plus Rhubarb Decoction)

*Gui Zhi Da Huang Tang* is a decoction of *Shao Yao* (Radix Paeoniae Lactiflorae), *Gan Cao* (Radix Glycyrrhizae), *Da Zao* (Fructus Zizyphi Jujubae), and *Jiang* (Rhizoma Zingiberis). It is used to cure the *tai yin* (pattern of cold damage) with abdominal fullness and pain and constipation.

*Da Chai Hu Tang* (Major Bupleurum Decoction)

*Da Chai Hu* includes *Ban Xia* (Rhizoma Pinelliae Ternatae), *Huang Qin* (Radix Scutellariae Baicalensis), and *Shao Yao* (Radix Paeoniae Lactiflorae), which quiet the spleen channel, and *Da Huang* (Radix Et Rhizoma Rhei) and *Zhi Shi* (Fructus Immaturus Citri Aurantii). It resolves (the exterior) as well as frees the flow of and moves (the interior).

*Xiao Cheng Qi Tang* (Minor Order the Qi Decoction)

*Xiao Cheng Qi* is composed of *Da Huang* (Radix Et Rhizoma Rhei), *Hou Po* (Cortex Magnoliae Officinalis), and *Zhi Shi* (Fructus Immaturus Citri Aurantii). It relieves hard stools and glomus fullness in the chest through moderate precipitation.

*Da Cheng Qi Tang* (Major Order the Qi Decoction)

---

[19] According to the author, this decoction seems to be composed of only one ingredient, *Huang Lian* (Rhizoma Coptidis Chinensis), but, to the best of the translator's knowledge, it is composed of *Huang Qin* (Radix Scutellariae Baicalensis), *Huang Lian* (Rhizoma Coptidis Chinensis), *Sheng Di* (uncooked Radix Rehmanniae), *Zhi Mu* (Rhizoma Anemarrhenae Aspheloidis), and *Gan Cao* (Radix Glycyrrhizae).

*Da Cheng Qi Tang* (Major Order the Qi Decoction)
*Da Cheng Qi* is composed of four ingredients, *Mang Xiao* (Mirabilitum), *Da Huang* (Radix Et Rhizoma Rhei), *Zhi Shi* (Fructus Immaturus Citri Aurantii), and *Hou Po* (Cortex Magnoliae Officinalis). It may relieve the pathocondition of glomus, fullness, dry, solid (stools), and tidal fever.

*Li Zhong Tang* (Rectify the Center Decoction)

*Li Zhong Tang* is composed of *Bai Zhu* (Rhizoma Atractylodis Macrocephalae), *Ren Shen* (Radix Panacis Ginseng), *Pao Jiang* (blast-fried Rhizoma Zingiberis), and *Zhi Gan Cao* (mix-fried Radix Glycyrrhizae). It cures the disease of vomiting, diarrhea, and abdominal pain with a deep pulse and cold qi (in the abdomen).

*Gui Zhi Ren Shen Tang* (Cinnamon Twig & Ginseng Decoction)

*Gui Zhi Ren Shen* includes *Gan Cao* (Radix Glycyrrhizae), *Bai Zhu* (Rhizoma Atractylodis Macrocephalae), and *Gan Jiang* (dry Rhizoma Zingiberis). It is able to cure cold in the center, generalized fever, abdominal pain, and diarrhea.

*Si Ni Tang* (Four Counterflows Decoction)

*Si Ni Tang* is composed of *Fu Zi* (Radix Lateralis Praeparatus Aconiti Carmichaeli), *Pao Jiang* (blast-fried Rhizoma Zingiberis), and *Zhi Gan Cao* (mix-fried Radix Glycyrrhizae). (In case of) a cold pattern with a deep, faint pulse, it may help the three *yang* become effulgent.

*Ma Huang Fu Zi Xi Xin Tang* (Ephedra, Aconite & Asarum Decoction)

*Ma Huang Fu Zi Xi Xin Tang* is a formula for direct stroke to the *shao yin* which manifests as a deep pulse, generalized fever, fear of cold, and a somber facial complexion.

*Gui Zhi Fu Zi Tang* (Cinnamon Twig & Aconite Decoction)

*Gui Zhi Fu Zi Tang* is composed of three flavors, (including) *Zhi Gan Cao* (mix-fried Radix Glycyrrhizae). With *Jiang* (Rhizoma Zingiberis) and *Da Zao* (Fructus Zizyphi Jujubae) added, it is a good formula for *shao yin* (pattern) headache and generalized aching.

*Huang Qi Jian Zhong Tang* (Astragalus Fortify the Center Decoction)

*Huang Qi Jian Zhong Tang* is a good formula for checking perspiration. It includes *Gui Zhi* (Ramulus Cinnamomi Cassiae), *Gan Cao* (Radix Glycyrrhizae), *Shao Yao* (Radix Paeoniae Lactiflorae), *Jiang* (Rhizoma Zingiberis), *Da Zao* (Fructus Zizyphi Jujubae), and *Yi Tang* (Maltose).

*Xiao Ban Xia Jia Fu Ling Tang* (Minor Pinellia Plus Poria Decoction)

*Ban Xia Fu Ling Tang* is a good formula for the pathocondition of water collecting below the heart. One should pound *Sheng Jiang* (uncooked Rhizoma Zingiberis), extract its juice, and put that in (the decoction). One dose is enough to effect a cure.

*Fu Zi Xie Xin Tang* (Aconite Drain the Heart Decoction)

*Fu Zi Xie Xin Tang* includes *Huang Qin* (Radix Scutellariae Baicalensis), *Huang Lian* (Rhizoma Coptidis Chinensis), and *Da Huang* (Radix Et Rhizoma Rhei). It is a remedy for aversion to cold, uncheckable sweating, and glomus below the heart.

*Xiao Xian Xiong Tang* (Minor Falling Chest Decoction)

*Xiao Xian Xiong* is a decoction of *Huang Lian* (Rhizoma Coptidis Chinensis), *Gua Lou* (Fructus Trichosanthis Kirlowii), and *Ban Xia* (Rhizoma Pinelliae Ternatae). It relieves chest binding which gives pain when pressed, eliminates fever, and removes phlegm drool.

*Da Xian Xiong Tang* (Major Falling Chest Decoction)

*Da Xian Xiong* is composed of *Gan Sui* (Radix Euphorbiae Kansui), *Mang Xiao* (Mirabilitum), and *Da Huang* (Radix Et Rhizoma Rhei). These (medicinals) all descend (*i.e.*, precipitate). Taking it immediately abates unbearable major binding.[20]

*Huang Lian Jie Du Tang* (Coptis Resolve Toxins Decoction)

*Huang Lian Jie Du Tang* is a good formula composed of four (ingredients), including *Zhi Zi* (Fructus Gardeniae Jasminoidis), *Huang Qin* (Radix Scutellariae Baicalensis), and *Huang Bai* (Cortex Phellodendri). If *Da Huang* (Radix Et Rhizoma Rhei) is added, it can remove heat toxins to cure *jue yin* (pattern) hemafecia and mania.

*Hua Ban Tang* (Transform Macules Decoction)

For macular eruption with vexation, agitation, and thirst, one should use *Hua Ban Tang*. It includes *Shi Gao* (Gypsum) and *Zhi Mu* (Rhizoma Anemarrhenae Aspheloidis) combined with *Xi Jiao* (Cornu Rhinocerotis) and *Yuan Shen* (Radix Scrophulariae Ningpoensis).

*Yin Chen Hao Tang* (Capillaris Decoction)

*Yin Chen Hao* is the best for cold damage with generalized yellowing. It includes *Da Huang* (Radix Et Rhizoma Rhei) and *Zhi Zi* (Fructus Gardeniae Jasminoidis). Once the flow of urine is freed and disinhibited, recovery follows.

*Tao Ren Cheng Qi Tang* (Persica Order the Qi Decoction)

*Tao Ren Cheng Qi Tang* treats blood amassment conditions such as mania. It includes *Gui Zhi* (Ramulus Cinnamomi Cassiae), *Gan Cao* (Radix

---

[20] This term implies the major chest binding pattern which manifests as hardness, fullness, and severe pain from below the heart down to the lower abdomen.

Glycyrrhizae), *Mang Xiao* (Mirabilitum), and *Da Huang* (Radix Et Rhizoma Rhei).

*Zhi Shi Zhi Zi Tang* (Aurantium Immaturus & Gardenia Decoction)

In this decoction, there are *Zhi Zi* (Fructus Gardeniae Jasminoidis), *Dou Chi* (Semen Praeparatus Sojae), and *Zhi Shi* (Fructus Immaturus Citri Aurantii). These three flavors are very strong (at eliminating heat). This is a good formula able to cure taxation with recurrent fever.

*Wen Dan Tang* (Warm the Gallbladder Decoction)

*Wen Dan Tang* is *Er Chen Tang* (Two Aged [Ingredients] Decoction) expanded by *Zhu Ru* (Caulis Bambusae In Taeniis) and *Zhi Shi* (Fructus Immaturus Citri Aurantii). It quiets and tranquilizes vacuity vexation causing insomnia after disease.

*Dang Gui Si Ni Tang* (Dang Gui Four Counterflows Decoction)

(This formula is composed of) *Dang Gui* (Radix Angelicae Sinensis), *Tong Cao* (Medulla Tetrapanacis Papyriferi), *Gan Cao* (Radix Glycyrrhizae), *Gui Zhi* (Ramulus Cinnamomi Cassiae), *Shao Yao* (Radix Paeoniae Lactiflorae), *Xi Xin* (Herba Asari Cum Radice), and *Da Zao* (Fructus Zizyphi Jujubae). If there is enduring cold internally, add *Sheng Jiang* (uncooked Rhizoma Zingiberis) and *Wu Zhu Yu* (Fructus Evodiae Rutecarpae).

*San Huang Shi Gao Tang* (Three Yellows Gypsum Decoction)

(This formula is composed of) *Huang Qin* (Radix Scutellariae Baicalensis), *Huang Bai* (Cortex Phellodendri), *Huang Lian* (Rhizoma Coptidis Chinensis), *Zhi Zi* (Fructus Gardeniae Jasminoidis), *Ma Huang* (Herba Ephedrae), *Dou Chi* (Semen Praeparatus Sojae), and *Shi Gao* (Gypsum Fibrosum).

*Wu Ling San* (Poria Five [Ingredients] Powder)

(This formula is composed of) *Bai Zhu* (Rhizoma Atractylodis Macrocephalae), *Ze Xie* (Rhizoma Alismatis), *Zhu Ling* (Sclerotium Polypori Umbellati), *Fu Ling* (Sclerotium Poriae Cocos), and *Gui Zhi* (Ramulus Cinnamomi Cassiae).

*Xiao Ban Qing Dai Yin* (Disperse Macules Indigo Drink)

(This formula is composed of) *Qing Dai* (Pulvis Indigonis), *Zhi Zi* (Fructus Gardeniae Jasminoidis), *Huang Lian* (Rhizoma Coptidis Chinensis), *Xi Jiao* (Cornu Rhinocerotis), *Zhi Mu* (Rhizoma Anemarrhenae Asphodeloidis), *Yuan Shen* (Radix Scrophulariae Ningpoensis), *Sheng Di* (uncooked Radix Rehmanniae), *Shi Gao* (Gypsum Fibrosum), *Chai Hu* (Radix Bupleuri), *Ren Shen* (Radix Panacis Ginseng), *Gan Cao* (Radix Glycyrrhizae), *Jiang* (Rhizoma Zingiberis), and *Da Zao* (Fructus Zizyphi Jujubae).

*Hui Yang Ji Jiu Tang* (Recover Yang Emergency Decoction)

*Hui Yang Ji Jiu* includes *Liu Jun* (Six Gentlemen [Decoction])[21], the group of flavors (consisting of) *Rou Gui* (Cortex Cinnamomi Cassiae), *Fu Zi* (Radix Lateralis Praeparatus Aconiti Carmichaeli), *Gan Jiang* (dry Rhizoma Zingiberis), and *Wu Wei Zi* (Fructus Schisandrae Chinensis), and three *li*[22] of *She Xiang* (Secretio Moschi Moschiferi) or (pig's) gall. This (formula) can accomplish an unusual feat in treating the three yin (patterns) with cold reversal.

*Qiang Huo Chong He Tang* (Notopterygium Harmonious Flow Decoction) [i.e., *Jiu Wei Qiang Huo Tang*, Nine Flavors Notopterygium Decoction; see the following subchapter]

---

[21] Six Gentlemen Decoction is composed of *Ren Shen* (Radix Panacis Ginseng), *Bai Zhu* (Rhizoma Atractylodis Macrocephalae), *Fu Ling* (Sclerotium Poriae Cocos), *Chen Pi* (Pericarpium Citri Reticulatae), *Gan Cao* (Radix Glycyrrhizae), and *Ban Xia* (Rhizoma Pinelliae Ternatae).

[22] One *li* equals 0.5 grams.

*Gui Zhi Jia Shao Yao Tang* (Cinnamon Twig Plus Peony Decoction) [*i.e., Gui Zhi Tang,* Cinnamon Twig Decoction with large amounts of *Shao Yao,* Radix Paeoniae Lactiflorae]

# 4. For Scourge Epidemic Disease, One Must First Be Clear About the Contraction & Offense of the Four Qi

Dan-xi said:

> If it is cold in spring when it should be warm, if it is cool in summer when it should be hot, if it is hot in autumn when it should be cool, and if it is warm in winter when it should be cold, this is untimely qi counter to the season. It is the reason why people old and young alike contract the same disease in the same year. This disease is called scourge epidemic.

At the beginning, the disease displays abhorrence of cold, vigorous fever, headache, generalized pain, thirst, and no aversion to wind cold. Its treatment is to effuse the exterior with *Ren Shen Bai Du San* (Ginseng Vanquish Toxins Powder) and to harmonize (the exterior and interior) with *Xiao Chai Hu Tang* (Minor Bupleurum Decoction). If an interior condition is observed, prescribe *Da Chai Hu Tang* (Major Bupleurum Decoction) to precipitate.

*Ren Shen Bai Du San* (Ginseng Vanquish Toxins Powder)

*Bai Du San* (Vanquish Toxins Powder) includes *Ren Shen* (Radix Panacis Ginseng), *Fu Ling* (Sclerotium Poriae Cocos), *Qian Hu* (Radix Peucedani), *Qiang Huo* (Radix Et Rhizoma Notopterygii), *Chai Hu* (Radix Bupleuri), and *Du Huo* (Radix Angelicae Pubescentis). Besides, there are *Jie Geng* (Radix Platycodi Grandiflori), *Chuan Xiong* (Radix Ligustici Wallichii), *Gan Cao* (Radix Glycyrrhizae), *Zhi Ke* (Fructus Citri Aurantii), *Bo He* (Herba Menthae Haplocalysis), and *Sheng Jiang* (uncooked Rhizoma Zingiberis). *Jiu Wei Qiang Huo Tang* (Nine Flavors Notopterygium Decoction)

*Jiu Wei Qiang Huo Tang* includes *Chuan Xiong* (Radix Ligustici Wallichii), *Xi Xin* (Herba Asari Cum Radice), *Bai Zhi* (Radix Angelicae Dahuricae),

*Gan Cao* (Radix Glycyrrhizae), *Fang Feng* (Radix Ledebouriellae Divaricatae), *Cang Zhu* (Rhizoma Atractylodis), *Huang Qin* (Radix Scutellariae Baicalensis), and *Sheng Di* (uncooked Radix Rehmanniae). It is a remedy for warm and febrile disease.

*Qin Lian Xiao Du San* (Scutellaria & Coptis Disperse Toxins Powder)

*Qin Lian Xiao Du San* includes *Gan Cao* (Radix Glycyrrhizae), *Jie Geng* (Radix Platycodi Grandiflori), *She Gan* (Rhizoma Belamcandae Diffusae), *Chuan Xiong* (Radix Ligustici Wallichii), *Fang Feng* (Radix Ledebouriellae Divaricatae), *Lian Qiao* (Fructus Forsythiae Suspensae), *Chai Hu* (Radix Bupleuri), *Jing Jie* (Herba Schizonepetae Tenuifoliae), *Bai Zhi* (Radix Angelicae Dahuricae), and *Zhi Ke* (Fructus Citri Aurantii). This is a formula for massive head (scourge) with sore pharynx (*i.e.*, throat).[23]

*Bing Jie San* (Resolve Ice Powder)

*Bing Jie San* is the best formula for simultaneously (causing) sweating and precipitation. It is composed of *Gui Xin* (Cortex Rasus Cinnamomi Cassiae),[24] *Gan Cao* (Radix Glycyrrhizae), *Bai Shao* (Radix Albus Paeoniae Lactiflorae), *Huang Qin* (Radix Scutellariae Baicalensis), *Ma Huang* (Herba Ephedrae), and *Da Huang* (Radix Et Rhizoma Rhei).

---

[23] Although Wiseman gives larynx for *yan* and pharynx for *hou*, either term is commonly used to refer to the throat in general. Massive head scourge refers to epidemic parotitis which is typically accompanied by sore throat.

[24] Cortex Rasus Cinnamomi Cassiae refers to the shaved bark of Cinnamon.

# 5. For Internal Damage of the Spleen & Stomach, One Should Identify Superabundance & Insufficiency

Dong-yuan[25] said:

> Lack of discipline in eating and drinking leads to stomach disease. When the stomach is diseased, the qi is short and essence spirit is scanty. When the stomach is vacuous, fire evils will (take the opportunity) to overwhelm it, generating great heat. From time to time, apparent fire ascends burning the face. The *Huang Di Zhen Jing (The Yellow Emperor's Classic of Needling)*[26] says, "Heat in the face is a foot *yang ming* disease." Once the stomach is diseased, the spleen has no place from which to receive its endowment and, therefore, also becomes diseased. (Conversely,) taxation and toil of the physical body results in spleen disease. When the spleen is diseased, there is fatigue and somnolence, loss of use of the limbs, and diarrhea. When the spleen is diseased, the stomach is not able by itself to move fluids and humors. Therefore, it also becomes diseased. In general, when the spleen and stomach are vacuous and weak, yang qi is not able to generate and grow. This is (known as) spring and summer failing to exercise their government. (For that reason,) the qi of the five viscera is not engendered. When the spleen is diseased, (the spleen qi) will flow downward to overwhelm the kidneys. Since earth restrains water, the bones become forceless. This is bone wilting. It causes the (sick) person's bone marrow to be empty and vacuous and unable to walk with their feet. This is doubling of yin qi, a pattern of yin exuberance with yang vacuity. The appropriate treatment is to upbear and invigorate yang with *Bu Zhong Yi Qi Tang* (Supplement the Center & Boost Qi Decoction).

Internal damage of the spleen and stomach: This may be detriment and damage done by hunger or overeating. Internal damage may also be a result of taking drastic medicinals. Because there are various different kinds (of internal damage), it should be treated with different methods.

---

[25] A.k.a. Li Gao (1180-1251 CE), one of the so-called Four Great Masters of the Jin-Yuan dynasties, whose main teaching was to emphasize the role of the spleen and stomach in pathology and treatment.

[26] I.e., the *Ling Shu (The Spiritual Pivot)*.

*Bu Zhong Yi Qi Tang* (Supplement the Center & Boost the Qi Decoction)

*Bu Zhong Yi Qi Tang* is composed of eight flavors: *Ren Shen* (Radix Panacis Ginseng), *Huang Qi* (Radix Astragali Membranacei), *Gan Cao* (Radix Glycyrrhizae), *Bai Zhu* (Rhizoma Atractylodis Macrocephalae), *Dang Gui* (Radix Angelicae Sinensis), *Sheng Ma* (Rhizoma Cimicifugae), *Chai Hu* (Radix Bupleuri), and *Chen Pi* (Pericarpium Citri Reticulatae). It is valuable when there is an insufficiency pattern.

*Jia Wei Ping Wei San* (Added Flavors Calm the Stomach Powder)

*Ping Wei San* is composed of *Shen Qu* (Massa Medica Fermentata), *Mai Ya* (Fructus Germinatus Hordei Vulgaris), *Cang Zhu* (Rhizoma Atractylodis), *Hou Po* (Cortex Magnoliae Officinalis), *Chen Pi* (Pericarpium Citri Reticulatae), *Gan Cao* (Radix Glycyrrhizae), *Mu Xiang* (Radix Auklandiae Lappae), *Shan Zha* (Fructus Crataegi), and *Cao Guo* (Fructus Amomi Tsao-ko). One dose and the intestines are loosened.[27]

*Ge Hua Jie Cheng Tang* (Pueraria Flower Resolve Hangover Decoction)

*Jie Cheng Tang* is composed of *Fu Ling* (Sclerotium Poriae Cocos), *Qing Pi* (Pericarpium Citri Reticulatae Viride), *Gan Jiang* (dry Rhizoma Zingiberis), *Bai Zhu* (Rhizoma Atractylodis Macrocephalae), *Chen Pi* (Pericarpium Citri Reticulatae), *Mu Xiang* (Radix Auklandiae Lappae), *Sha Ren* (Fructus Amomi), *Ren Shen* (Radix Panacis Ginseng), *Shen Qu* (Massa Medica Fermentata), *Dou Kou* (Fructus Cardamomi), *Ze Xie* (Rhizoma Alismatis), *Ge Hua* (Flos Puerariae), and *Zhu Ling* (Sclerotium Polypori Umbellati).

# 6. In External Contraction of Febrile Disease, One Should Know Summerheat From Spring Warmth

Nowadays, people speak of diseases of fever as four seasons cold damage, but few know about the theory of the exit and entrance (of evils). In

---

[27] Loosening the intestines means precipitating food accumulation and relieving abdominal pain.

wintertime, cold evils enter (the body) from outside. Therefore, one should use a heavy formula of *Ma Huang* (Herba Ephedrae), *Gui Zhi* (Ramulus Cinnamomi Cassiae), (etc.) to promote sweating. In spring and summer, the pathocondition of fever may be due to contraction of cold in winter. However, it does not cause an outbreak (then). Rather, cold toxins are treasured within the skin and muscles (*i.e.*, flesh). When spring comes, these transform into warm disease, and, when summer comes, they transform into febrile disease. Since these evils come out from within, one should use a light formula of *Qiang Huo* (Radix Et Rhizoma Notopterygii), *Qian Hu* (Radix Peucedani), (etc.) to resolve the exterior.

If one contracts sudden untimely cold in the spring, summer, or autumn, it is appropriate to take formulas which course the exterior and free the flow of qi, such as *Xiang Su Yin* (Cyperus & Perilla Drink), *Shen Su Yin* (Ginseng & Perilla Drink), and *Shi Shen Tang* (Ten Spirits Decoction).

*Shi Shen Tang* (Ten Spirits Decoction)

*Shi Shen Tang* is composed of *Ge Gen* (Radix Puerariae), *Chuan Xiong* (Radix Ligustici Wallichii), *Bai Zhi* (Radix Angelicae Dahuricae), *Chi Shao* (Radix Rubrus Paeoniae Lactiflorae), *Zi Su* (Folium Perillae Frutescentis), *Chen Pi* (Pericarpium Citri Reticulatae), *Ma Huang* (Herba Ephedrae), *Sheng Ma* (Rhizoma Cimicifugae), *Xiang Fu* (Rhizoma Cyperi Rotundi), and *Zhi Gan Cao* (mix-fried Radix Glycyrrhizae). It treats flu and (other) epidemics.

*Shen Su Yin* (Ginseng & Perilla Drink)

*Shen Su Yin* includes *Er Chen Tang* (Two Aged [Ingredients] Decoction) with *Zhi Ke* (Fructus Citri Aurantii), *Jie Geng* (Radix Platycodi Grandiflori), *Ge Gen* (Radix Puerariae), *Qian Hu* (Radix Peucedani), and *Mu Xiang* (Radix Auklandiae Lappae). This is a prescription for coughing of phlegm in the four seasons. It is good for (patterns) with no sweating.

*Xiang Su Yin* (Cyperus & Perilla Drink)

[See #3, present chapter.]

# 7. Sudden Wind Stroke Has Four Causes & Is Classified as Three Categories in Terms of Treatment

In the *Qian Jin Fang (Prescriptions [Worth] A Thousand [Pieces] of Gold)*, there are four major species of wind stroke. They are known as hemilateral withering[28] or hemiplegia, wind disablement or loss of use of the limbs with no generalized pain, wind choke or sudden inability to recognize people, and wind impediment, which looks like wind (*i.e.*, rheumatoid arthritis).

Liu He-jian[29] said:

> Wind stroke paralysis is not due to stroke of external wind but is entirely to inappropriate ways of health care. (As a result,) heart fire becomes fulminantly effulgent and the kidney water becomes vacuous and exhausted so as not to restrain (heart fire). Then yin becomes vacuous, and yang replete. Heat qi is depressed so that the heart and spirit are clouded, and the use of the sinews and bones is lost. There may arise sudden collapse with loss of consciousness.

Dong-yuan said:

> (In terms of) wind stroke, the wind evils do not come from outside. As a mater of fact, this is a disease of the qi. The qi of people over 40 years old is debilitated. If, at such an age, anxiety, joy, indignation, or anger damage the qi, they are liable to have this disease. At a robust age, it does not happen. Occasionally, (however,) fat, exuberant persons may be taken with it. This, too, is due to qi debility in spite of an exuberant physical form.

Dan-xi said:

> In the southeast, the qi is warm and the ground is usually damp. There, wind disease is not (a disease of) wind. It is always ascribed to dampness

---

[28] Although Wiseman gives desiccation for *ku*, we believe that here withering makes more sense, since this condition is not just a drying out but a wilting and atrophy.

[29] A.k.a. Liu Wan-su (1120-1200 CE), one of the so-called Four Great Masters of the Jin-Yuan dynasties. He was the founder of the Cool & Cold (Medicinals) School, and his theory eventually led to the establishment of the warm disease school.

which engenders phlegm. Phlegm engenders heat, and heat engenders wind.

In the *Fa Ming Lun (Treatise Making Clear [the Study of Medicine])*[30], it says that the condition of wind stroke is divided into bowel stroke, visceral stroke, and blood vessel stroke. Bowel stroke usually involves the limbs, (manifesting) an ashen facial complexion (literally, a face colored like earth), a floating pulse, aversion to wind cold, and hypertonicity and insensitivity of the limbs. (Wind) stroke involving either the front or the back or the side of the body is called bowel stroke. This is usually easy to cure. In visceral stroke, obstruction usually occurs to the nine orifices. Slack lips, loss of voice, deafness, nasal congestion, distorted vision, and urinary and fecal stoppage are all called visceral stroke. They are usually difficult to treat. Blood vessel stroke manifests as deviated mouth and eyes.

The above three categories are treated in different ways. Suppose blood vessel stroke is complicated by an external pathocondition of the six channels. (The treatment in that case) should be based on *Xiao Xu Ming Tang* (Minor Prolong Destiny Decoction) to effuse the exterior, incorporating an acrid, cool formula like *Tong Sheng San* (Sage-communicated [*i.e.*, inspired] Powder). Suppose bowel stroke is complicated by urinary and fecal block internally. (The treatment) should be based on *San Hua Tang* (Three Transformations Decoction) to attack the interior. However, one should avoid carrying out diaphoresis and precipitation beyond measure. Overdoing diaphoresis leads to yang collapse, and overdoing precipitation to collapse of yin. Collapse of yang is the same as detriment of the defensive, and collapse of yin is the same as detriment of the constructive. One should never be careless about this. If there is no pathocondition of the six channels externally and no urinary and fecal block internally, but there is paralysis of the hand and foot and difficult, sluggish speech, this is stroke to the channels and network vessels. In that case, it is appropriate to supplement the blood and to nourish the sinews with *Da Qin Jiao Tang* (Major Gentian Macrophylla

---

[30] A medical work by Li Gao, a.k.a. Li Dong-yuan.

Decoction) and *Qiang Huo Yu Feng Tang* (Notopterygium Cure Wind Decoction).

(In case of) wind stroke of phlegm reversal, coma, sudden collapse, and unconsciousness of human affairs, one may first roll powdered *Zao Jiao* (Fructus Gleditschiae Chinensis) in paper, burn it, and blow the smoke into the (patient's) nose. If this succeeds in provoking snorting, (the condition) is treatable. If not, it is difficult to treat. After that, one may use a phlegm-ejection formula: Administer five *fen* of powdered *Zao Jia* (Fructus Gleditschiae Chinensis) and five *fen* of finely powdered *Bai Fan* (Alumen) mixed with *Jiang Zhi* (Succus Rhizomatis Zingiberis), and then apply mechanical ejection.[31] (Finally,) administer *Dao Tan Tang* (Abduct Phlegm Decoction).

Hemiplegia is called paralysis. In general it is caused by streaming of phlegm drool. If it is treated without delay at the early stage, it may be alright, but, over time, phlegm fire will be depressed and bound up, and any prescriptions scarcely bring effect.

For deviated mouth and eyes with no complications, use equal amounts of powdered *Bai Fu Zi* (Rhizoma Typhonii Gigantei), *Jiang Can* (Bombyx Batryticatus), and *Quan Xie* (Buthus Martensi) [all used uncooked]. Take two *qian* each time with wine. This is called *Qian Zheng San* (Correct Deviation Powder). Another method is to use one *liang* of *Bi Ma Zi Rou* (Semen Rinici Communis) and three *fen* of *Bing Pian* (Borneol). Pound these together into a paste. This is called *Gai Rong Gao* (Correct the Looks Paste). In cold months, add one *qian* each of *Jiang* (Rhizoma Zingiberis) and *Fu Zi* (Radix Lateralis Praeparatus Aconiti Carmichaeli). In case of left deviation, apply the paste to the right side. In case of right deviation, apply it to the left side. It is also effective to apply blood of *Shan Yu* (Monopterus Albus) and *Bing Pian* (Borneol).

For wind stroke with stiff tongue impeding speech, use *Qing Dai* (Pulvis Indigonis), *Peng Sha* (Borax), and *Bo He* (Herba Menthae Haplocalysis),

---

[31] In modern clinical practice, Chinese doctors do not adopt ejection, etc. to treat wind stroke for fear these methods may endanger the life of such a patient.

two *qian* each, and *Bing Pian* (Borneol) and *Niu Huang* (Calculus Bovis), three *fen* each. Powder them finely. First, wash the tongue with diluted honey, and then rub it with ginger juice. Finally, mix the (above) medicinals with honey and apply (this mixture) over the tongue.

For wind stroke with clenched jaws, it is appropriate to rub the gums with *Wu Mei Rou* (Fructus Pruni Mume). When the gums become sore and soft, (the mouth) will open easily. Or mix powdered *Li Lu* (Radix Et Rhizoma Veratri) with a small amount of *She Xiang* (Secretio Moschi Moschiferi). Mix five *fen* of this with water, and then pour into the nose to provoke ejection.

*Xiao Xu Ming Tang* (Minor Prolong Destiny Decoction)

*Xu Ming Tang* is composed of *Gui Zhi* (Ramulus Cinnamomi Cassiae), *Ma Huang* (Herba Ephedrae), *Ren Shen* (Radix Panacis Ginseng), *Chuan Xiong* (Radix Ligustici Wallichii), *Fang Feng* (Radix Ledebouriellae Divaricatae), *Fu Zi* (Radix Lateralis Praeparatus Aconiti Carmichaeli), *Huang Qin* (Radix Scutellariae Baicalensis), *Xing Ren* (Semen Pruni Armeniacae), *Gan Cao* (Radix Glycyrrhizae), *Bai Shao* (Radix Albus Paeoniae Lactiflorae), and *Fang Ji* (Radix Stephanae Tetrandrae). Turn to this (formula) in case of wind stroke of the blood vessels.

Appendix: *Xu Ming Tang* (Prolong Destiny Decoction) in the *Gu Jin Lu Yan (Proven Formulas Recorded From Ancient to Modern Times)*[32]

(This is composed of) *Ma Huang* (Herba Ephedrae), *Gui Zhi* (Ramulus Cinnamomi Cassiae), *Dang Gui* (Radix Angelicae Sinensis), *Ren Shen* (Radix Panacis Ginseng), *Shi Gao* (Gypsum Fibrosum), *Gan Jiang* (dry Rhizoma Zingiberis), *Gan Cao* (Radix Glycyrrhizae), *Chuan Xiong* (Radix Ligustici Wallichii), and *Xing Ren* (Semen Pruni Armeniacae).

*Fang Feng Tong Sheng San* (Ledebouriella Sage-communicated Powder)

---

[32] A formulary composed by Zhen Li-yan of the Tang dynasty (*circa* 540-620 CE).

*Tong Sheng San* is composed of *Jing Jie* (Herba Schizonepetae Tenuifoliae), *Fang Feng* (Radix Ledebouriellae Divaricatae), *Lian Qiao* (Fructus Forsythiae Suspensae), *Ma Huang* (Herba Ephedrae), *Gan Cao* (Radix Glycyrrhizae), *Bo He* (Herba Menthae Haplocalysis), *Dang Gui* (Radix Angelicae Sinensis), *Zhi Zi* (Fructus Gardeniae Jasminoidis), *Huang Qin* (Radix Scutellariae Baicalensis), *Chuan Xiong* (Radix Ligustici Wallichii), *Jie Geng* (Radix Platycodi Grandiflori), *Bai Zhu* (Rhizoma Atractylodis Macrocephalae), *Shi Gao* (Gypsum Fibrosum), *Bai Shao* (Radix Albus Paeoniae Lactiflorae), *Hua Shi* (Talcum), *Mang Xiao* (Mirabilitum), and *Da Huang* (Radix Et Rhizoma Rhei).

*San Hua Tang* (Three Transformations Decoction)

This is *Xiao Cheng Qi Tang* (Minor Order the Qi Decoction) plus *Qiang Huo* (Radix Et Rhizoma Notopterygii).

*Da Qin Jiao Tang* (Major Gentiana Macrophylla Decoction)

*Da Qin Jiao* is *Ba Zhen Tang* (Eight Pearls Decoction) minus *Ren Shen* (Radix Panacis Ginseng) and plus *Xi Xin* (Herba Asari Cum Radice), *Huang Qin* (Radix Scutellariae Baicalensis), *Qiang Huo* (Radix Et Rhizoma Notopterygii), *Du Huo* (Radix Angelicae Pubescentis), *Shi Gao* (Gypsum Fibrosum), *Bai Zhi* (Radix Angelicae Dahuricae), and *Fang Feng* (Radix Ledebouriellae Divaricatae). It dispels wind as well as nourishes yin.

*Dao Tan Tang* (Abduct Phlegm Decoction)

[See chapter 11 above.]

*Qiang Huo Yu Feng Tang* (Notopterygium Cure Wind Decoction)

(This is composed of) *Qiang Huo* (Radix Et Rhizoma Notopterygii), *Du Huo* (Radix Angelicae Pubescentis), *Fang Feng* (Radix Ledebouriellae Divaricatae), *Fang Ji* (Radix Stephaniae Tetrandae), *Chai Hu* (Radix Bupleuri), *Qian Hu* (Radix Peucedani), *Ma Huang* (Herba Ephedrae), *Xi Xin* (Herba Cum Radice Asari), *Bai Zhi* (Radix Angelicae Dahuricae), *Ju Hua* (Flos Chrysanthemi Morifolii), *Bo He Ye* (Folium Menthae

Haplocalysis), *Qin Jiao* (Radix Gentianae Macrophyllae), *Man Jing Zi* (Fructus Viticis), *Dang Gui* (Radix Angelicae Sinensis), *Chuan Xiong* (Radix Ligustici Wallichii), *Shu Di* (prepared Radix Rehmanniae), *Zhi Gan Cao* (mix-fried Radix Glycyrrhizae), *Huang Qi* (Radix Astragali Membranacei), *Zhi Ke* (Fructus Citri Aurantii), *Di Gu Pi* (Cortex Radicis Lycii Chinensis), *Ren Shen* (Radix Panacis Ginseng), *Zhi Mu* (Rhizoma Anemarrhenae Asphodeloidis), *Gou Qi Zi* (Fructus Lycii Chinensis), carbonized *Du Zhong* (Cortex Eucommiae Ulmoidis), and ginger-processed *Ban Xia* (Rhizoma Pinelliae Ternatae), two *liang* each; *Guan Gui* (tubiform Cortex Cinnamomi Cassiae), one *liang; Fu Ling* (Sclerotium Poriae Cocos) and *Huang Qin* (Radix Scutellariae Baicalensis), three *liang* each; *Sheng Di* (uncooked Radix Rehmanniae), *Cang Zhu* (Rhizoma Atractylodis), *Shi Gao* (Gypsum Fibrosum), and *Shao Yao* (Radix Paeoniae Lactiflorae), four *liang* each. Make coarse powder of all the above medicinals and administer one *liang* each time. Decoct in water and administer.

# 8. There Are Three Categories of Breaking & Damaging Wind and Its Treatment Is Based on the Division of Three Channels

The pattern of breaking and damaging wind may be caused by wind which takes advantage of knocks and falls to settle (in the body) or by wind evils which take the opportunity of sores refusing to close for a long time to assault (the body). It may also be the result of bathing or washing with hot water or being moxaed. The qi of hot water or (moxa) fire does the same work as wind evils. The symptoms include alternating fever and chills, and, if extreme, clenched jaws, deviated eyes, and rigidity of the body. It may cause death any time and is very dreadful.

If the pulse is floating and forceless, this is a *tai yang* (pattern). It may be cured through diaphoresis. If the pulse is long and forceful, this is a *yang ming* (pattern). Precipitation may cure it. If the pulse is floating, bowstring, and small, this is a *shao yang* (pattern). Harmonization (of the exterior and interior) may effect a cure. Once (evils) have transmitted into the interior, there is no way to cure it.

*Qiang Huo Fang Feng Tang* (Notopterygium & Ledebouriella Decoction)

*Qiang Huo Fang Feng Tang* includes *Chuan Xiong* (Radix Ligustici Wallichii), *Gan Cao* (Radix Glycyrrhizae), *Gao Ben* (Radix Et Rhizoma Ligustici Chinensis), *Dang Gui* (Radix Angelicae Sinensis), *Xi Xin* (Herba Asari Cum Radice), *Di Yu* (Radix Sanguisorbae Officinalis), and *Bai Shao* (Radix Albus Paeoniae Lactiflorae). Taking it may effect recovery if (evils) are in the exterior.

*Yu Zhen San* (True Jade Powder)

Prepare and powder equal amounts of *Fang Feng* (Radix Ledebouriellae Divaricatae) and *Nan Xing* (Rhizoma Arisaematis). First, apply them to the affected part, and then take two *qian* brewed in warm wine. This also treats rabid dog bite.

# 9. Summerheat Stroke Has Stirring & Still Varieties

After the summer solstice, heat disease is summerheat (disease). Zhang Jie-gu[33] said, "Stirring and then stroke is called sunstroke, while stillness and then stroke is called summerheat stroke." Dong-yuan said, "Stroke during taxation and toil is called sunstroke, while stroke when sheltering indoors from summerheat called summerheat stroke." The disease of sunstroke is caused by taxation and toil in the open and exposure of the skin to the sun. Heat qi invades through the nostrils and damages the lung channel. The symptoms include generalized fever, headache, shivering with goose flesh, slight (aversion to) cold, mouth kept open, dry teeth, (the presence of) tongue fur, and vexatious thirst. The appropriate treatment is *Ren Shen Shi Gao Zhi Mu Tang* (Ginseng, Gypsum & Anemarrhena Decoction). While staying quietly in the house or walking in the streets, if one is suddenly subjected to fuming and steaming of depressive heat and breathes in summerheat qi, the pericardium may be damaged. The symptoms include vexatious thirst, spontaneous sweating,

---

[33] A.k.a. Zhang Yuan-su, a preeminent physician during the Jin Dynasty (1115-1234 CE), teacher of many distinguished physicians of that time, including Li Gao.

a facial complexion as if covered with dirt, and a vacuous pulse. There may (also) possibly be abdominal pain and diarrhea or retching, agitation, and oppression. In extreme (cases), there is clouding (of the spirit) with inability to recognize people. The appropriate treatment is *Xiang Ru Yin* (Elsholtzia Beverage).

*Ren Shen Shi Gao Zhi Mu Tang* (Ginseng, Gypsum & Anemarrhena Decoction)

(This formula is composed of) *Shi Gao* (Gypsum Fibrosum), *Zhi Mu* (Rhizoma Anemarrhenae Asphodeloidis), *Gan Cao* (Radix Glycyrrhizae), *Ren Shen* (Radix Panacis Ginseng), and *Jing Mi* (Semen Oryzae Sativae).

*Xiang Ru Yin* (Elsholtzia Drink)

*Xiang Ru Yin* includes *Hou Po* (Cortex Magnoliae Officinalis), *Bian Dou* (Semen Dolichoris Lablab), and a pinchful of *Huang Lian* (Rhizoma Coptidis Chinensis). (It treats) summerheat stroke with abdominal pain, vomiting, and diarrhea due to contention between yin and yang.[34]

*Shi Wei Xiang Ru Yin* (Ten Flavors Elsholtzia Drink)

*Shi Wei Xiang Ru Yin* includes *Ren Shen* (Radix Panacis Ginseng), *Huang Qi* (Radix Astragali Membranacei), *Bai Zhu* (Rhizoma Atractylodis Macrocephalae), *Fu Ling* (Sclerotium Poriae Cocos), *Chen Pi* (Pericarpium Citri Reticulatae), *Hou Po* (Cortex Magnoliae Officinalis), *Gan Cao* (Radix Glycyrrhizae), *Mu Gua* (Fructus Chaenomelis Lagenariae), and *Bian Dou* (Semen Dolichoris Lablab). It clears summerheat and fortifies the spleen channel.

*Liu He Tang* (Six Harmonies Decoction)

*Liu He* is composed of *Fu Ling* (Sclerotium Poriae Cocos), *Bai Zhu* (Rhizoma Atractylodis Macrocephalae), *Ren Shen* (Radix Panacis Ginseng),

---

[34] Contention between yin and yang means disharmony between the defensive and constructive. In other words, there is a mixed yin-yang or exterior-interior pattern.

*Xiang Ru* (Herba Elsholtziae Seu Moslae), *Huo Xiang* (Herba Agastachis Seu Pogostemi), *Bian Dou* (Semen Dolichoris Lablab), *Sha Ren* (Fructus Amomi), *Ban Xia* (Rhizoma Pinelliae Ternatae), *Gan Cao* (Radix Glycyrrhizae), *Mu Gua* (Fructus Chaenomelis Lagenariae), *Xing Ren* (Semen Pruni Armeniacae), and *Hou Po* (Cortex Magnoliae Officinalis). (It treats) sudden turmoil with summerheat damaging the spirit.[35]

*Sheng Mai San* (Engender the Pulse Powder)

*Sheng Mai San* is composed of *Ren Shen* (Radix Panacis Ginseng), *Wu Wei Zi* (Fructus Schisandrae Chinensis), and *Mai Dong* (Tuber Ophiopogonis Japonici). It clears the heart, eliminates heat from the lungs, supplements the qi, and generates fluids.

*Qing Shu Yi Qi Tang* (Clear Summerheat & Boost the Qi Decoction)

*Yi Qi Tang* is composed of *Dang Gui* (Radix Angelicae Sinensis), *Huang Qi* (Radix Astragali Membranacei), *Ju Pi* (Pericarpium Citri Reticulatae), *Bai Zhu* (Rhizoma Atractylodis Macrocephalae), *Cang Zhu* (Rhizoma Atractylodis), *Gan Cao* (Radix Glycyrrhizae), *Qing Pi* (Pericarpium Citri Reticulatae Viride), *Huang Bai* (Cortex Phellodendri), *Ren Shen* (Radix Panacis Ginseng), *Mai Dong* (Tuber Ophiopogonis Japonici), *Wu Wei Zi* (Fructus Schisandrae Chinensis), *Sheng Ma* (Rhizoma Cimicifugae), *Ge Gen* (Radix Puerariae), *Shen Qu* (Massa Medica Fermentata), and *Ze Xie* (Rhizoma Alismatis).

# 10. Dampness Affection Is Divided into Internal & External

Dan-xi said, "Of the six qi, disease caused by damp heat amounts to eight or nine out of ten(cases)." (Damp heat) may be contracted from outside or produced by internal damage. If one lives in a damp environment in

---

[35] Sudden turmoil is the name of a disease characterized by sudden vomiting and diarrhea, such as cholera. Damaged spirit usually refers to mental disorders like listlessness and somnolence.

a low place, walks in mist and dew early in the morning, walks in the rain, wades in water, or wears sweat-soaked clothes and wet shoes, external dampness may be contracted. If one indulges in wine or overeats uncooked, chilled (foods), dampness may be contracted through internal damage. There is another theory saying that drink and food entering the stomach are none other but damp (substances). As long as spleen earth is effulgent, it is able to convey and transform water and grains, sending (the essence from these) up to the lungs and transporting it down to the urinary bladder. Then no damp qi can be retained. If the spleen is too weak to convey and transform water and grains, this, too, causes dampness.

As to the method of treating dampness, people in the past merely took water disinhibition as the ruling (principle). (However,) one should not adhere to one method. It is necessary to prescribe medicinals in accordance with the (particular) pathocondition. If damp qi is in the skin, the appropriate medicinals are those that resolve the exterior, such as *Ma Huang* (Herba Ephedrae), *Gui Zhi* (Ramulus Cinnamomi Cassiae), *Fang Ji* (Radix Stephaniae Tetrandae), *Cang Zhu* (Rhizoma Atractylodis), and *Bai Zhu* (Rhizoma Atractylodis Macrocephalae). This is analogous to sullenness of the six ways.[36] (The weather) cannot clear except after it has rained.

If water dampness accumulates in the stomach and intestines causing swelling and distention of the abdomen, the appropriate medicinals are those which attack and precipitate, such as *Da Huang* (Radix Et Rhizoma Rhei), *Gan Sui* (Radix Euphorbiae Kansui), *Da Ji* (Herba Seu Radix Cirsii Japonici), *Yuan Hua* (Flos Daphnes Genkwae), *Qian Niu* (Semen Pharbiditis), and *Bing Lang* (Semen Arecae Catechu). This is likened to water flushing the ditches. It cannot be removed except through conducting.

If cold dampness is in the skin, flesh, sinews, and bones giving rise to hypertonicity and contracting pain or insensitivity, the appropriate medicinals are channel-warming ones like *Gan Jiang* (dry Rhizoma

---

[36] The six ways include heaven, earth, and the four quarters, east, west, south, and north. This phrase means sullen sky or weather.

Zingiberis), *Fu Zi* (Radix Lateralis Praeparatus Aconiti Carmichaeli), *Ding Xiang* (Flos Caryophylli), and *Rou Gui* (Cortex Cinnamomi Cassiae). This is likened to the sun hanging in the sky which must certainly dry up yin dampness.

If damp qi lies between the viscera and bowels and the skin and flesh and it is slight, not serious, the appropriate medicinals are those of fortifying the spleen and drying dampness, such as *Cang Zhu* (Rhizoma Atractylodis), *Bai Zhu* (Rhizoma Atractylodis Macrocephalae), *Hou Po* (Cortex Magnoliae Officinalis), *Ban Xia* (Rhizoma Pinelliae Ternatae), *Mu Xiang* (Radix Auklandiae Lappae), and *Sang Pi* (Cortex Radicis Mori Albi). This is likened to a small amount of dampness requiring only ash or earth to absorb it. Then the dampness will certainly be dried.

If damp heat lies in the lower abdomen or the urinary bladder, giving rise to swelling, diarrhea, or urinary block, it is appropriate to use percolating and draining medicinals like *Zhu Ling* (Sclerotium Polypori Umbellati), *Ze Xie* (Rhizoma Alismatis), *Fu Ling* (Sclerotium Poriae Cocos), *Hua Shi* (Talcum), *Yin Chen* (Herba Artemisiae Capillaris), *Mu Tong* (Caulis Akebiae), *Ting Li* (Semen Lepidii Seu Descurainiae), *Che Qian Zi* (Semen Plantaginis), and *Hai Jin Sha* (Spora Lygodii Japonici). This is likened to water flooding the ditches which cannot flow away except when the outlets are dredged.

If damp qi lies in the skin, it is appropriate to use medicinals for vanquishing water, such as *Fang Feng* (Radix Ledebouriellae Divaricatae), *Qiang Huo* (Radix Et Rhizoma Notopterygii), and *Du Huo* (Radix Angelicae Pubescentis). This is likened to a fresh breeze sending crisp air which must certainly disperse damp qi.

# 11. Fire Has Seven Types

Dan-xi said,

> The five phases each have one nature except for fire which is classified into two — sovereign fire and ministerial fire. Sovereign fire is the heart fire,

and ministerial fire is the life gate fire. (The latter) fire comes from the former heaven.

In addition, there are the fires of the five minds.[37] When violent anger gives rise to qi counterflow, fire arises in the liver. When sorrow and grief stir the center, fire arises in the lungs. When intoxication and overeating cause (internal) damage, fire arises in the spleen. Excessive sexual activity may give rise to fire in the kidneys. Excessive thought and preoccupation may give rise to fire in the heart. These fires are produced by people themselves.

Disease caused by fire involves not only the five viscera and the twelve channels. Whenever there is superabundant qi, there is fire. All wind with shaking and dizzy vision, rib-side pain, and red eyes are ascribed to stirring liver fire. (For them,) *Chai Hu* (Radix Bupleuri) and *Huang Lian* (Rhizoma Coptidis Chinensis) are the ruling medicinals. All pain, sores, and mouth and tongue sores are ascribed to stirring heart fire. (For them,) *Huang Lian* (Rhizoma Coptidis Chinensis) is the ruling medicinal. All dampness with swelling and distention, mouth sores, and bad breath are ascribed to stirring spleen fire. (For this,) *Shao Yao* (Radix Paeoniae Lactiflorae) is the ruling medicinal. All qi rushing depression, dry cough, and nosebleeding are ascribed to stirring lung fire. (For this,) *Zhi Zi* (Fructus Gardeniae Jasminoidis) and *Huang Qin* (Radix Scutellariae Baicalensis) are the ruling medicinals. Seminal emission, dream emission, and red and white urinary turbidity are ascribed to stirring kidney fire. (For this,) *Zhi Mu* (Rhizoma Anemarrhenae Asphodeloidis) is the ruling medicinal.

Yellow eyes, a bitter (taste) in the mouth, and restlessness when either sitting or lying down are ascribed to stirring gallbladder fire. (For this,) *Chai Hu* (Radix Bupleuri) is the ruling medicinal. Dribbling urinary block, dripping, and red and white vaginal discharge and turbidity are ascribed to stirring small intestine fire. (For this,) *Mu Tong* (Caulis Akebiae) is the

---

[37] Previously, Wiseman translated *zhi* as orientation. Other translators use the modern Chinese usage of will. In this case, mind should be understood as a synonym for affect or emotion.

ruling medicinal. Toothache, gaping gums, and swollen cheeks and jowls are ascribed to stirring stomach fire. (For this,) *Shi Gao* (Gypsum Fibrosum) is the ruling medicinal. (The presence of) tongue fur, sore throat, and constipation are ascribed to stirring large intestine fire. (For this,) *Huang Qin* (Radix Scutellariae Baicalensis) and *Da Huang* (Radix Et Rhizoma Rhei) are the ruling medicinals. Inhibited urination and lower abdominal pain are ascribed to stirring bladder fire. (For this,) *Huang Bai* (Cortex Phellodendri) is the ruling medicinal. Dizzy head, fatigue, and heat in the palms and soles of the feet are ascribed to stirring triple burner fire. (For this,) *Chai Hu* (Radix Bupleuri) and *Huang Qin* (Radix Scutellariae Baicalensis) are the ruling medicinals. Frequent erection and incessant seminal emission are ascribed to stirring life gate fire. (For this,) *Huang Bai* (Cortex Phellodendri) is the ruling medicinal. All the above are bitter, cold medicinals which can drain superabundant fire.

According to the *Yu Ji Wei Yi* (*The Subtle Meanings of the Jade Mechanism*)[38], if there is food damage, taxation damage, internal damage of the original qi, spontaneous sweating, fever, and fatigue, and if the pulse is large and forceless, the qi opening being two or three times as large as man's prognosis[39], this is a pattern of yang vacuity. To relieve it, one should prescribe sweet, warm medicinals like *Huang Qi* (Radix Astragali Membranacei), *Ren Shen* (Radix Panacis Ginseng) and *Gan Cao* (Radix Glycyrrhizae).

With yin faint and yang strong, ministerial fire is so effulgent as to overwhelm the yin phase, stewing (yin)[40] day after day. This is a pattern

---

[38] Its original name was *Yi Xue Zhe Zhong* (*Compromise in the Study of Medicine*) written by Xu Yong-cheng (?-1380 CE). This is an outstanding medical work embracing nearly every branch of Chinese medicine.

[39] The right inch position of the wrist pulse is sometimes called the qi opening, while the left inch position is also called the *ren ying* or man's prognosis. The pulse at the Adams apple is also called *ren ying*.

[40] Stewing yin implies growing emaciation and decrease in fluids, for example, dry mouth.

of blood vacuity. The appropriate medicinals are yin-enriching ones like *Di Huang* (Radix Rehmanniae), *Tian Men Dong* (Tuber Asparagi Cochinensis), *Huang Bai* (Cortex Phellodendri), *Yuan Shen* (Radix Scrophulariae Ningpoensis), *Gui Ban* (Plastrum Testudinis), *Dang Gui* (Radix Angelicae Sinensis), *Zhi Mu* (Rhizoma Anemarrhenae Asphodeloidis), *Wu Wei* (Fructus Schisandrae Chinensis), *Suo Yang* (Herba Cynomorii Songarici), *Niu Xi* (Radix Achyranthis Bidentatae), and *Hu Gu* (Os Trigridis). These are taken in pill form.

If heart fire is extremely hyperactive with depressed heat repletion internally, this is a pattern of yang overpowering. To overcome it, one may use cold, salty medicinals like *Da Huang* (Radix Et Rhizoma Rhei) and *Mang Xiao* (Mirabilitum).

When kidney water is damaged with true yin losing its guard (*i.e.*, not controlling yang), this is rootless fire, a pattern of yin vacuity. To treat it, one should use water-invigorating medicinals like *Sheng Di* (uncooked Radix Rehmanniae) and *Yuan Shen* (Radix Scrophulariae Ningpoensis).

If life gate fire is debilitated, this is yang collapse disease. There will be impotence and inability to take in food. The right cubit pulse is slow, thin, and forceless. When there is no fire in the life gate, this is like no fuel under the cauldron. To treat this, one may use warm and hot medicinals like *Fu Zi* (Radix Lateralis Praeparatus Aconiti Carmichaeli) and *Gan Jiang* (dry Rhizoma Zingiberis).

If the stomach is vacuous, overeating uncooked, chilled foods may cause yang qi to be suppressed within spleen earth. This is a pattern of fire depression. (To treat it,) one should use upbearing and dissipating medicinals to effuse it, such as *Sheng Ma* (Rhizoma Cimicifugae) and *Ge Gen* (Radix Puerariae).

## 12. Phlegm Has Ten Causes

Phlegm cannot engender itself, and, whenever it is engendered, there must be some cause, possibly cold, possibly heat, possibly dampness, possibly summerheat, possibly dryness, possibly wine accumulation, possibly food accumulation, possibly spleen vacuity, possibly kidney vacuity. Nowadays, when people treat phlegm, they know only phlegm-treating medicinals like *Nan Xing* (Rhizoma Arisaematis) and *Ban Xia* (Rhizoma Pinelliae Ternatae) but do not know how to treat the root of phlegm. As a result, even more phlegm is generated and the disease becomes even more difficult to eliminate.

As for myself, I have only an imperfect knowledge, but I venture to give an account of the medicinals of treating the root. If phlegm is generated by wind, the phlegm that is expectorated is foamy and the pulse is floating and bowstring. To treat this, use *Qian Hu* (Radix Peucedani), *Xuan Fu Hua* (Flos Inulae), and the like. If phlegm is generated by cold, the phlegm that is expectorated is clear and cold and the pulse is slow and deep. To treat this, use *Jiang* (Rhizoma Zingiberis), *Gui Zhi* (Ramulus Cinnamomi Cassiae), *Xi Xin* (Herba Asari Cum Radice), and the like. If phlegm is generated by heat, the phlegm that is expectorated is sticky and yellow and the pulse is surging and rapid. To treat this, use *Huang Qin* (Radix Scutellariae Baicalensis), *Huang Lian* (Rhizoma Coptidis Chinensis), *Zhi Zi* (Fructus Gardeniae Jasminoidis), *Shi Gao* (Gypsum Fibrosum), and the like. If phlegm is generated from dampness, the phlegm that is expectorated is jade-green and the pulse is floating and moderate. To treat this, use *Cang Zhu* (Rhizoma Atractylodis), *Fu Ling* (Sclerotium Poriae Cocos), and the like. If phlegm is generated by summerheat, the phlegm that is expectorated smells fishy and the pulse is vacuous and faint. To treat this, use *Xiang Ru* (Herba Elsholtziae Seu Moslae), *Bian Dou* (Semen Dolichoris Lablab), and the like. If phlegm is generated by dryness, the phlegm that is expectorated is like a thread, globules, or sticky lacquer. The phlegm is difficult to hack out and the pulse is slippery and rapid. To treat this, use *Lou Ren* (Semen Trichosanthis Kirlowii), *Hua Fen* (Semen Trichosanthis Kirlowii), *Bei Mu* (Bulbus Fritillariae), and the like. If phlegm is generated from wine accumulation, phlegm is expectorated with retching and nausea and, in the morning, coughing. To treat this, use *Zhu Ling* (Sclerotium Polypori Umbellati), *Ge Hua* (Flos Puerariae), and the like. If phlegm is generated from food accumulation, the phlegm that is expectorated is like peach gelatin or shaped like a clam and there is oppression and discomfort in the chest and abdomen. To treat this, use *Xiang Fu* (Rhizoma Cyperi Rotundi), *Zhi Shi* (Fructus Immaturus Citri Aurantii), *Shen Qu* (Massa Medica Fermentata), *Mai Ya* (Fructus Germinatus Hordei Vulgaris), and the like. If phlegm is generated by spleen vacuity, there will be frequent expectoration of phlegm, fatigue, and reduced eating. To treat this, use *Bai Zhu* (Rhizoma Atractylodis Macrocephalae), *Chen Pi* (Pericarpium Citri Reticulatae), and the like. If phlegm is generated by kidney vacuity, once phlegm is (begun to be) expectorated out, it will be like tides swelling. This arises during the fifth watch.[41] To treat this, use *Tian Men Dong* (Tuber Asparagi Cochinensis), *Mai Men Dong* (Tuber Ophiopogonis Japonici), *Wu Wei Zi* (Fructus Schisandrae Chinensis), and the like.

All the above medicinals, however, serve only as adjuvants or assistants. The ruling formula is *Er Chen Tang* (Two Aged [Ingredients] Decoction) which is indispensable in any case.

*Er Chen Tang* (Two Aged [Ingredients] Decoction) [See chapter 11 above.]

*Dao Tan Tang* (Abduct Phlegm Decoction) [See chapter 11 above.]

*Gun Tan Wan* (Roll Phlegm Pills)

*Gun Tan Wan* is composed of *Da Huang* (Radix Et Rhizoma Rhei) and *Huang Qin* (Radix Scutellariae Baicalensis), one half catty each, *Qing Meng Shi* (Lapis Micae Seu Chloriti), one *liang*, and five *qian* of good quality *Kui Chen* (Lignum Aquilariae Agallochae).

# 13. The Qi Has Nine Problems

The qi is the ruler of the entire body. As long as there is no damage by the seven affects internally and no offence by cold or summerheat externally, the qi flows freely around (the body), visiting all the hundreds of bones.

---

[41] *I.e.*, around dawn.

If there is interference by the seven affects or offence by cold or summerheat, then disease will arise.

It is said in the *Nei Jing (Inner Classic)* that:

> Anger causes the qi to rise, joy causes the qi to slacken, sorrow causes the qi to disperse, fear causes the qi to descend, fright causes the qi to be chaotic, taxation leads to qi consumption, thought causes the qi to bind, cold causes the qi to contract, and heat causes the qi to drain. These nine qi differ from each other and (thus) cause different (kinds of) diseases.

Zhang Zi-he[42] has given a detailed discussion about this. I need not recount it again.

In terms of qi vacuity and qi repletion, repletion means repletion of evil qi, while vacuity means vacuity of righteous qi. If qi vacuity is the cause of disease, then various (kinds of) diseases, (such as) lack of essence spirit, fatigue and somnolence, reduced eating, dizziness, crippling wilt, spontaneous sweating, diarrhea, seminal emission, or prolapse (of the rectum), may arise. After examining the pathocondition and the pulse, if one verifies qi vacuity, one ought to use *Ren Shen* (Radix Panacis Ginseng), *Huang Qi* (Radix Astragali Membranacei), *Bai Zhu* (Rhizoma Atractylodis Macrocephalae), and the like.

If there is heart pain, rib-side pain, or lower abdominal qi pain, then there is evil qi obstruction and nonmovement of the righteous qi. They are responsible for these pains. What is evil qi? It may be cold, heat, phlegm, food, or blood. The (treatment) principle is first to remove the evils. Then the righteous qi will flow freely and pain stops. Generally speaking, qi is categorized as yang and, to regulate the qi, one must use warm, dissipating medicinals such as *Chen Xiang* (Lignum Aquilariae Agallochae), *Mu Xiang* (Radix Auklandiae Lappae), *Ding Xiang* (Flos Caryophylli), *Hui Xiang* (Fructus Foeniculi Vulgaris), *Bai Dou Kou* (Fructus

---

[42] A.k.a. Zhang Cong-zheng (1156-1228 CE), one of the so-called Four Great Masters of the Jin-Yuan dynasties, founder of School of Attacking & Precipitating.

Cardamomi), *Chen Pi* (Pericarpium Citri Reticulatae), *Xiang Fu* (Rhizoma Cyperi Rotundi), and *Sha Ren* (Fructus Amomi).

If disease has endured for days and this has led to qi transforming into fire, one cannot prescribe warm, hot medicinals alone. One must use *Huang Qin* (Radix Scutellariae Baicalensis), *Huang Lian* (Rhizoma Coptidis Chinensis), *Zhi Zi* (Fructus Gardeniae Jasminoidis), and the like as the ruling (ingredients) and small amounts of hot medicinals as conductors.

There is another point of view that the qi is the precursor of the blood, while the blood is the spouse of the qi. (Therefore,) when the qi is diseased, the blood cannot remain disinhibited alone and also becomes diseased. For that reason, to medicinals for treating the qi, one should add blood-rectifying medicinals like *Dang Gui* (Radix Angelicae Sinensis), *Shao Yao* (Radix Paeoniae Lactiflorae), *Chuan Xiong* (Radix Ligustici Wallichii), *Hong Hua* (Flos Carthami Tinctorii), and *Tao Ren* (Semen Pruni Persicae).

## 14. Depression Has Six Names

Dan-xi said:

> So long as the qi and blood enjoy harmonious flow, none of the hundreds of diseases can arise. Once they are depressed and suppressed, various diseases are produced.

In general, depression is part of any disease. If depression endures, it will generate disease, or, if a disease has endured, depression will be generated. Therefore, to treat any disease, one has to take depression into account in the treatment scheme.

There are six categories of depression: qi, blood, dampness, heat, food, and phlegm. Qi depression manifests as chest and rib-side pain and a deep, choppy pulse. Blood depression manifests as lack of strength in the four limbs, ability to take in food, reddish stools, and a deep pulse. Dampness depression manifests as migratory pain around the body or pain in the joints that starts in wet and cold (weather), and a deep, thin and moderate pulse. Heat depression manifests as visual distortion, oppression, reddish urine, and a deep, rapid pulse. Food depression manifests as acid belching, (persistent) satiety and fullness, and no liking of food. The man's prognosis pulse is normal, but the qi opening pulse is exuberant. Phlegm depression manifests as panting and fullness arising on movement and a deep, slippery pulse in the inch opening.

To treat these, use *Liu Yu Tang* (Six Depressions Decoction) and *Yue Ju Wan* (Out-thrust Tribulation Pills) as the ruling formulas. In case of dampness, add *Bai Zhu* (Rhizoma Atractylodis Macrocephalae) and *Qiang Huo* (Radix Et Rhizoma Notopterygii). In case of qi, add *Mu Xiang* (Radix Auklandiae Lappae) and *Bing Lang* (Semen Arecae Catechu). In case of food, add *Shan Zha* (Fructus Crataegi) and *Sha Ren* (Fructus Amomi). In case of blood, add *Tao Ren* (Semen Pruni Persicae) and *Hong Hua* (Flos Carthami Tinctorii). In case of heat, add *Chai Hu* (Radix Bupleuri) and *Huang Qin* (Radix Scutellariae Baicalensis). In case of phlegm, add *Ban Xia* (Rhizoma Pinelliae Ternatae) and *Nan Xing* (Rhizoma Arisaematis).

*Liu Yu Tang* (Six Depressions Decoction)

*Liu Yu* is composed of *Xiang Fu* (Rhizoma Cyperi Rotundi), *Cang Zhu* (Rhizoma Atractylodis), *Shen Qu* (Massa Medica Fermentata), *Zhi Zi* (Fructus Gardeniae Jasminoidis), *Lian Qiao* (Fructus Forsythiae Suspensae), *Zhi Ke* (Fructus Citri Aurantii), *Chen Pi* (Pericarpium Citri Reticulatae), *Chuan Xiong* (Radix Ligustici Wallichii), *Huang Qin* (Radix Scutellariae Baicalensis), *Su Geng* (Caulis Perillae Frutescentis), and *Gan Cao* (Radix Glycyrrhizae). It is able to soothe all types of depression and binding.

*Yue Ju Wan* (Out-thrust Tribulation Pills)

*Yue Ju Wan* opens depression. It is composed of *Xiang Fu* (Rhizoma Cyperi Rotundi), *Cang Zhu* (Rhizoma Atractylodis), *Chuan Xiong* (Radix Ligustici Wallichii), *Zhi Zi Ren* (Fructus Gardeniae Jasminoidis) and *Shen Qu* (Massa Medica Fermentata), all in equal amounts. In case of dampness, add *Bai Zhu* (Rhizoma Atractylodis Macrocephalae) and *Fu Ling* (Sclerotium Poriae Cocos). In case of heat, add *Qing Dai* (Pulvis Indigonis). In case of phlegm, add *Nan Xing* (Rhizoma Arisaematis), *Hai Shi* (Pumice), and *Gua Lou* (Fructus Trichosanthis Kirlowii). In case of blood, add *Tao Ren* (Semen Pruni Persicae) and *Hong Hua* (Flos Carthami Tinctorii). In case of food, add *Shan Zha* (Fructus Crataegi) and *Sha Ren* (Fructus Amomi). In case of qi, add *Mu Xiang* (Radix Auklandiae Lappae).

## 15. Malaria Is Due to Assailment by Summerheat Wind, but May Be Complicated by Phlegm & Food

The *Nei Jing (Inner Classic)* says, "If summerheat causes damage in summer, then malaria will arise in autumn." It also says:

Cold (*i.e.*, shivering) preceding heat (*i.e.*, fever), is called cold malaria. Heat preceding cold is called warm malaria. If there is solely heat without cold, it is called pure-heat malaria.

Dan-xi said:

There are summerheat malaria, wind malaria, warm malaria, phlegm malaria, and food malaria. If the evils lie in the qi division, it will start soon. If the evils lie in the blood division, it will start slowly (*i.e.*, take a long time to start). In addition, (malaria) may persist long with the evil qi hidden in the rib-side where it is bound into a concretion lump. This is known as mother of malaria.

In malaria, the typical pulse is bowstring. If the pulse is rapid as well as bowstring, there is abundant heat. If it is slow as well as bowstring, there is abundant cold. If it is bowstring and short, there is food damage. If it is bowstring and slippery, there is abundant phlegm. If it is faint, there is vacuity. If it is regularly interrupted and scattered, (the condition) is dangerous.

If, during the attack of malaria, deafness, rib-side pain, alternating fever and chills, a bitter taste in the mouth, and frequent retching arise and the pulse is bowstring, this is usually wind malaria, (requiring) *Xiao Chai Hu Tang* (Minor Bupleurum Decoction). If, during the attack of malaria, there is more heat than cold, a bitter (taste) in the mouth, dry throat, difficult voidings of reddish urine, and a bowstring, rapid pulse, this is usually yang malaria, (requiring) *Qing Pi Yin* (Clear the Spleen Beverage). If, during the attack of malaria, heat precedes cold, this is usually warm malaria, (requiring) *Shi Gao Zhi Mu Tang* (Gypsum & Anemarrhena Decoction) plus *Gui Zhi* (Ramulus Cinnamomi Cassiae). If, during the attack of malaria, there is solely heat without cold, this is called pure heat malaria. It should be impugned to summerheat. Either *Xiang Ru Yin* (Elsholtzia Beverage) plus *Fu Ling* (Sclerotium Poriae Cocos) or *Chai Hu Shi Gao Zhi Mu Tang* (Bupleurum, Gypsum & Anemarrhena Decoction) is good (for it). If, during the attack of malaria, there is solely cold without heat and the pulse is slow, this is called male malaria.[43] It should be impugned to cold, (requiring) *Shu Qi San* (Dichroa Powder).

If, during the attack of malaria, there is pain all over the body with heaviness of the arms and legs and more cold than heat and the pulse is soggy, this is called damp malaria, (requiring) *Chai Ping Tang* (Bupleurum Calm [the Stomach] Decoction). If (malaria) is caused by epidemic pestilential qi and during the attack there is sometimes cold and sometimes heat with generalized heaviness, this is called miasmic malaria, (requiring) *Ping Wei San* (Calm the Stomach Powder) plus *Huo Xiang* (Herba Agastachis Seu Pogostemi), *Shi Chang Pu* (Rhizoma Acori Graminei), and *Sheng Jiang* (uncooked Rhizoma Zingiberis). If malaria is with abundant phlegm and chest fullness, during its attack there are clouding, restlessness, and raving, and the pulse is bowstring and slippery, this is called phlegm malaria, (requiring) *Er Cheng Tang* (Two Aged [Ingredients] Decoction) plus *Chang Shan* (Radix Dichroae Febrifugae), *Cao Guo* (Fructus Amomi Tsao-ko), *Huang Qin* (Radix Scutellariae Baicalensis), and *Chai Hu* (Radix Bupleuri).

Malaria with inhibited chest and diaphragm and aversion to the smell of food is food malaria. It requires *Qing Pi Yin* (Clear the Spleen Drink) plus *Shan Zha* (Fructus Crataegi), *Shen Qu* (Massa Medica Fermentata), and *Mai Ya* (Fructus Germinatus Hordei Vulgaris). Malaria with accumulation and stagnation causing chest fullness, more heat than cold, and dry, solid

---

[43] Cold is yin, white yin in turn often stands for females or women. Therefore this kind of malaria should be spoken of as female malaria.

stools (requires) *Da Chai Hu Tang* (Major Bupleurum Decoction) to precipitate (accumulation). Malarial disease with inability to bear the slightest taxation that persists all year round with frequent relapse is called taxation malaria. (It requires) *Xiao Chai Hu Tang* (Minor Bupleurum Decoction) with *Ban Xia* (Rhizoma Pinelliae Ternatae) removed and *Tian Hua Fen* (Radix Trichosanthis Kirlowii) added. Night malaria[44] requires abducting (the evils) into the yang division and, hence, dispersing them with blood medicinals, such as *Chuan Xiong* (Radix Ligustici Wallichii), *Dang Gui* (Radix Angelicae Sinensis), *Hong Hua* (Flos Carthami Tinctorii), *Cang Zhu* (Rhizoma Atractylodis), *Bai Zhi* (Radix Angelicae Dahuricae), *Huang Bai* (Cortex Phellodendri), and *Gan Cao* (Radix Glycyrrhizae). Decoct in water, expose them in the open for one night, and then administer.

For mother of malaria, use vinegar-fried *Bie Jia* (Carapax Amydae Sinensis), *San Leng* (Rhizoma Sparganii), *E Zhu* (Rhizoma Curcumae Zedoariae), *Mu Xiang* (Radix Auklandiae Lappae), *Xiang Fu* (Rhizoma Cyperi Rotundi), *Hai Shi* (Pumice), *Qing Pi* (Pericarpium Citri Reticulatae Viride), *Tao Ren* (Semen Pruni Persicae), *Hong Hua* (Flos Carthami Tinctorii), *Shen Qu* (Massa Medica Fermentata), and *Mai Ya* (Fructus Germinatus Hordei Vulgaris). Make these into pills with vinegar and administer with boiling water.

To interrupt malaria, use *Chang Shan* (Radix Dichroae Febrifugae), *Cao Guo* (Fructus Amomi Tsao-ko), *Bing Lang* (Semen Arecae Catechu), and *Zhi Mu* (Rhizoma Anemarrhenae Asphodeloidis), one *qian* each. Decoct in water, expose for one night, and administer warm during the fifth watch with a cup of hot wine.

*Xiao Chai Hu Tang* (Minor Bupleurum Decoction) [See chapter 12 above.]

*Qing Pi Yin* (Clear the Spleen Drink)

*Qing Pi Yin* is composed of *Chai Hu* (Radix Bupleuri), *Huang Qin* (Radix Scutellariae Baicalensis), *Gan Cao* (Radix Glycyrrhizae), *Hou Po* (Cortex

---

[44] This refers to malaria that attacks during the night.

Magnolia Officinalis), *Qing Pi* (Pericarpium Citri Reticulatae Viride), *Fu Ling* (Sclerotium Poriae Cocos), *Ban Xia* (Rhizoma Pinelliae Ternatae), *Bai Zhu* (Rhizoma Atractylodis Macrocephalae), and *Cao Guo* (Fructus Amomi Tsao-ko). Phlegm and food malaria will respond to it.

*Shi Gao Zhi Mu Tang* (Gypsum & Anemarrhena Decoction) [See #3 above.]

*Xiang Ru Yin* (Elsholtzia Drink) [See #9 above.]

*Chai Hu Shi Gao Zhi Mu Tang* (Bupleurum, Gypsum & Anemarrhena Decoction)

This is *Xiao Chai Hu Tang* (Minor Bupleurum Decoction) combined with *Shi Gao Zhi Mu Tang* (Gypsum & Anemarrhena Decoction).

*Shu Qi San* (Dichroa Powder)

Wash *Shu Qi* (Folium Dichroae) to clear its fishy smell. Burn *Yun Mu* (Muscovitum) for two days. Pound them together with *Long Gu* (Os Draconis) into powder. Take one half *qian* with boiled water towards the attack.

*Chai Ping Tang* (Bupleurum Calming [the stomach] Decoction)

This is *Xiao Chai Hu Tang* (Minor Bupleurum Decoction) combined with *Ping Wei San* (Calm the Stomach Powder).

*Er Chen Tang* (Two Aged [Ingredients] Decoction) [See chapter 11 above.]

*Ping Wei San* (Calm the Stomach Powder) [See chapter 13 above.]

*Da Chai Hu Tang* (Major Bupleurum Decoction) [See #3 above.]

# 16. The Causes of Dysentery Are Dampness, Heat and Accumulation & Collecting

Dysentery is a pathocondition of abdominal urgency (or cramping), rectal heaviness (*i.e.*, tenesmus), and blood or pus or mixed pus and blood (in the stools) with or without (abdominal) pain. The origin of this pathocondition is located in no other than three (causes): dampness, heat, and food accumulation. If these damage the qi division, dysentery precipitates white (pus). If they damage the blood division, dysentery precipitates red (blood). If they damage both the qi and the blood, there are mixed red and white (in the stools).

In regard to dysentery, if the pulse is faint and small, this is favorable. If it is floating and surging, this is unfavorable. If it is slippery and large, this is favorable. If it is bowstring and urgent (or tense), this is unfavorable.

Liu He-jian said, "(As for) the great methods of treating dysentery, moving the blood leads to pus in the stools being automatically cured, while regulating the qi automatically eliminates rectal heaviness." He also said:

Rectal heaviness should be precipitated, while abdominal should be harmonized. If there is generalized heaviness, it is necessary to remove dampness. If the pulse is bowstring, it is necessary to dispel wind. If pus and blood are thick and sticky, one should use heavy medicinals[45] to resolve (toxins). Generalized cold with spontaneous sweating requires hot medicinals to warm. If evil wind comes from outside (causing dysentery), this requires diaphoresis. If dysentery is like duck slop, this requires warming.

Proven methods for treating dysentery: At the onset of dysentery with pus and blood in the stools, abdominal urgency, and rectal heaviness, use *Shao Yao Tang* (Peony Decoction). For white dysentery, use *Wen Liu Wan*

---

[45] These are medicinals which are heavy in weight and have the function of precipitation as well as settling the spirit.

(Warm the Six [Bowels] Pills).[46] For red dysentery, use *Qing Liu Wan* (Clear the Six [Bowels] Pills). For red and white dysentery with abdominal urgency and rectal heaviness, use *Li Xiao San* (Powder of Instant Efficacy). If upbearing and astringing medicinals are used instead of precipitating ones at the onset of dysentery, this will lead to accumulation of miscellaneous evils internally and nonmovement of blood causing unbearable abdominal pain. Then use *Tao Ren Cheng Qi Tang* (Persica Order the Qi Decoction). If dysentery is complicated by fever, there is wind evils in the stomach and intestines. (To treat this,) decoct and administer *Ren Shen Bai Du San* (Ginseng Vanquish Toxins Powder) plus *Huang Lian* (Rhizoma Coptidis Chinensis), *Chen Cang Mi* (aged Semen Oryzae Sativae), *Sheng Jiang* (uncooked Rhizoma Zingiberis), and *Da Zao* (Fructus Zizyphi Jujubae). For epidemic dysentery prohibiting intake of food, add seven pieces of *Shi Lian Zi Rou* (Semen Caesalpiniae Minacis). If dysentery has persisted long with red and white (substances in the stools) already finished but there arises vacuity cold with prolapse of the rectum, use *Yang Zang Tang* (Nurture the Viscera Decoction).

*Shao Yao Tang* (Peony Decoction)

*Shao Yao Tang* (Peony Decoction) treats dysentery, curing rectal heaviness. It is composed of *Huang Qin* (Radix Scutellariae Baicalensis), *Huang Lian* (Rhizoma Coptidis Chinensis), *Rou Gui* (Cortex Cinnamomi Cassiae), *Da Huang* (Radix Et Rhizoma Rhei), *Mu Xiang* (Radix Auklandiae Lappae), *Bing Lang* (Semen Arecae Catechu), *Dang Gui* (Radix Angelicae Sinensis), and *Gan Cao* (Radix Glycyrrhizae).

*Wen Liu Wan* (Warm the Six [Bowels] Pills)

(This is composed of) *Hua Shi* (Talcum), six *liang*, ground in water; *Fen Cao* (debarked Radix Glycyrrhizae), one *liang*; and *Gan Jiang* (dry Rhizoma Zingiberis), five *qian*. Powder and make into pills with water.

---

[46] *Liu*(six) in the formula name means nothing more than there is an ingredient, *Hua Shi* (Talcum), which is six *liang* in amount.

*Qing Liu Wan* (Clear the Six [Bowels] Pills)

(This is composed of) *Hua Shi* (Talcum), six *liang*, ground in water; *Fen Cao* (debarked Radix Glycyrrhizae), one *liang*; and *Hong Qu* (Massa Medica Fermentata Cum Semenis Oryzam Sativam), five *qian*. Powder and make into pills with water.

*Li Xiao San* (Powder of Instant Efficacy)

(This is composed of) *Huang Lian* (Rhizoma Coptidis Chinensis), four *liang*, washed with wine; *Wu Zhu Yu* (Fructus Evodiae Rutecarpae), two *liang*, stir-frying the above two together and then removing the *Wu Zhu Yu*; *Chen Pi* (Pericarpium Citri Reticulatae), two *liang*; *Zhi Ke* (Fructus Citri Aurantii), two *liang*, bran-fried. Powder these together and take three *qian* per dose with Shaoxing wine. In case of dysentery prohibiting intake of food, take with thin gruel of *Chen Cang Mi* (aged Semen Oryzae Sativae).

*Tao Ren Cheng Qi Tang* (Persica Order the Qi Decoction) [See #3 above.]

*Ren Shen Bai Du San* (Ginseng Vanquish Toxins Powder) [See #4 above.]

*Yang Zang Tang* (Nurture the Viscera Decoction)

*Yang Zang* is composed of *Bai Shao* (Radix Albus Paeoniae Lactiflorae), *Dang Gui* (Radix Angelicae Sinensis), *Ren Shen* (Radix Panacis Ginseng), *Rou Gui* (Cortex Cinnamomi Cassiae), *Bai Zhu* (Rhizoma Atractylodis Macrocephalae), *Mu Xiang* (Radix Auklandiae Lappae), *Gan Cao* (Radix Glycyrrhizae), *Mi Ke* (Pericarpium Papaveris Somniferi), *He Zi* (Fructus Terminaliae Chebulae), *Rou Kou* (Semen Myristicae Fragrantis), and *Wu Mei* (Fructus Pruni Mume).

*He Zhong Tang* (Harmonize the Center Decoction)

*He Zhong* is composed of *Dang Gui* (Radix Angelicae Sinensis), wine-processed *Huang Lian* (Rhizoma Coptidis Chinensis), *Chen Pi* (Pericarpium Citri Reticulatae), *Bai Shao* (Radix Albus Paeoniae Lactiflorae), *Hou Po* (Cortex Magnoliae Officinalis), *Cang Zhu* (Rhizoma Atractylodis), *Gan Cao*

(Radix Glycyrrhizae), *Fu Ling* (Sclerotium Poriae Cocos), and *Zhi Ke* (Fructus Citri Aurantii). This cures both new and enduring dysentery.

## 17. Retching & Vomiting Is Caused by Counterflow of Stomach Qi Which Refuses to Descend

(Trying to vomit) with noise is called retching, while (expelling) substances is called vomiting. The noise is ascribed to qi and fire. The substances are phlegm and food. Interference by cold qi, summerheat stroke, indignation and anger causing qi counterflow, excessive wine and food causing damage, roundworms causing pain, enduring disease causing stomach vacuity, or accumulated phlegm and blood stasis are all capable of giving rise to retching and vomiting.

Generally speaking, if the pulse is vacuous and thin, this is favorable. If the pulse is replete and large, this is unfavorable.

For treatment, use *Er Chen Tang* (Two Aged [Ingredients] Decoction) as the ruling (formula). If there is cold in the stomach with inability to take in even water, while the pulse is deep and slow, add *Gan Jiang* (dry Rhizoma Zingiberis), *Rou Gui* (Cortex Cinnamomi Cassiae), *Ding Xiang* (Flos Caryophylli), *Yi Zhi* (Fructus Alpiniae Oxyphyllae), and the like. In case of summerheat damage with vexatious thirst, a dirty facial complexion, a vacuous pulse, and generalized fever, add *Huang Lian* (Rhizoma Coptidis Chinensis), *Bian Dou* (Semen Dolichoris Lablab), *Xiang Ru* (Herba Elsholtziae Seu Moslae), *Hou Po* (Cortex Magnolia Officinalis), and the like. Anger causes liver fire to surge against the stomach so as to give rise to retching, a bitter (taste) in the mouth, and inhibited chest and rib-side. The pulse is bowstring and rapid. (In that case,) add *Xiang Fu* (Rhizoma Cyperi Rotundi), *Shao Yao* (Radix Paeoniae Lactiflorae), *Huang Qin* (Radix Scutellariae Baicalensis), *Huang Lian* (Rhizoma Coptidis Chinensis), *Wu Mei* (Fructus Pruni Mume), *Zhu Ru* (Caulis Bambusae In Taeniis), and the like. In case of food damage causing vomiting of sour, foul matter, add *Shan Zha* (Fructus Crataegi), *Cao Guo* (Fructus Amomi Tsao-ko), *Shen Qu* (Massa Medica Fermentata), *Mai Ya* (Fructus Germinatus Hordei Vulgaris), *Zhi Shi* (Fructus Immaturus Citri Aurantii),

*Sha Ren* (Fructus Amomi), and the like. In case of retching and vomiting caused by drinking excessive wine damaging (the stomach), add *Ge Hua* (Flos Puerariae), *Zhu Ling* (Sclerotium Polypori Umbellati), *Ze Xie* (Rhizoma Alismatis), *Bai Dou Kou* (Fructus Cardamomi), and the like. In case of vomiting caused by upward assailment of roundworms, add *Wu Mei* (Fructus Pruni Mume), *Chuan Jiao* (Pericarpium Zanthoxyli Bungeani), *Huang Bai* (Cortex Phellodendri), *Gan Jiang* (dry Rhizoma Zingiberis), *Bai Zhu* (Rhizoma Atractylodis Macrocephalae), and the like. If enduring disease causes stomach vacuity and, hence, retching which arises on smelling grain qi, then add *Ren Shen* (Radix Panacis Ginseng), *Bai Zhu* (Rhizoma Atractylodis Macrocephalae), *Fu Long Gan* (Terra Flava Ustae), *Huo Xiang* (Herba Agastachis Seu Pogostemi), and the like. If phlegm accumulates in the stomach causing retching and vomiting, add *Nan Xing* (Rhizoma Arisaematis), *Zhi Shi* (Fructus Immaturus Citri Aurantii), *Zhu Ru* (Caulis Bambusae In Taeniis), *Jiang Zhi* (Succus Rhizomatis Zingiberis), and the like. If vomiting is caused by internal damage with blood stasis, add mashed *Tao Ren* (Semen Pruni Persicae), *Jiang Zhi* (Succus Rhizomatis Zingiberis), and the like.

(Once) a person had damage done by taking in excessive food. (They suffered from) abdominal pain, constipation, and incessant retching and vomiting. I thought, it is normal if the qi of the *yang ming* descends but abnormal if it keeps ascending. Therefore, in this case, retching and vomiting were due to constipation which made the stomach qi unable to descend. Based on this (understanding), precipitation was required. (I) prescribed *Pi Ji Wan* (Spleen Accumulation Pills). One dose effected recovery.

A person recovered from sudden turmoil of vomiting and diarrhea but began to suffer from vomiting on taking in food. (Food) was unable to stay (in the stomach for a moment). I said, vomiting and diarrhea are due to slippery qi. It was necessary to treat these with astringing medicinals. (I) prescribed *Shao Zhen Wan* (Burn the Needle Pills). Three doses effected recovery.

*Er Chen Tang* (Two Aged [Ingredients] Decoction) [See chapter 11 above.]

*Pi Ji Wan* (Spleen Accumulation Pills)

(This is composed of) *E Zhu* (Rhizoma Curcumae Zedoariae), *San Leng* (Rhizoma Sparganii), *Liang Jiang* (Rhizoma Alpiniae Officinari), *Qing Pi* (Pericarpium Citri Reticulatae Viride), *Mu Xiang* (Radix Auklandiae Lappae), *Bai Cao Shuang* (Pulvis Fumi Carbonisati), and mashed *Jiang Zi* (Semen Crotonis Tiglii). Grind into a mash and make into pills with flour. It is extraordinarily efficacious if taken with *Ju Pi Tang* (Orange Peel Decoction).

*Shao Zhen Wan* (Burn the Needle Pills)

(This is composed of) *Huang Dan* (Minium), ground in water; *Ku Bai Fan* (Alumen Praeparatum); and *Zhu Sha* (Cinnabar), all in equal amounts. Powder and make with dates into pills the size of Euryales seeds. Insert needles into the pills. Then (holding them by the needles), burn them with their nature preserved, and finally powder them. Take seven *fen* per dose with cool water or rice water.

# 18. Diarrhea Is Due to Damaged, Unbalanced Spleen Qi

Dan-xi said, "Diarrhea may be due to dampness, fire, qi vacuity, phlegm accumulation, or food accumulation." Dai Yuan-li[47] said by way of annotation:

> Watery diarrhea with no abdominal pain is due to dampness. Inability of food to stay in the stomach after entrance or nontransformation of food is due to qi vacuity. Abdominal pain with watery diarrhea and rumbling in the intestines, the abdominal pain being spasmodic and followed by diarrhea, is due to fire. (Sometimes) diarrhea and (sometimes) no diarrhea with the amounts of stools (sometimes) large and (sometimes) small is due

---

[47] A.k.a. Dai Si-gong (1324-1405 CE), pupil of Zhu Zhen-heng (Dan-xi) who is supposed to be the real writer of many works with Zhu Zhen-heng's name as the author.

to phlegm accumulation. Severe abdominal pain with diarrhea, the pain relieved by diarrhea, is due to food accumulation.

The disease of diarrhea may be contracted in different ways in the four seasons. It may be caused by the interference of wind, cold, summerheat or dampness or by drink and food damage. When the spleen and stomach qi is stirred up and damaged, diarrhea arises.

Its treatment should be different (depending upon whether) it is new or enduring and based on a study of its causes. If it is new (*i.e.*, recent onset), medicinals quelling evils should be the ruling ones with spleen-fortifying ones as assistants. If it is enduring, spleen-supplementing medicinals should sovereign while upbearing and effusing ones should be the envoys. Before prescribing medicinals, I always identify the pattern. Below is an account (of my prescriptions) that have proven to be reliable.

If what is precipitated is green and there is abdominal pain and a floating pulse, this is due to contained wind. One should, (therefore, use) *Qiang Huo* (Radix Et Rhizoma Notopterygii), *Fang Feng* (Radix Ledebouriellae Divaricatae), and the like. If what is precipitated is white and there is abdominal pain, a deep, slow, weak pulse, cold limbs, and clear urine, this is due to contained cold. One should, (therefore, use) *Gan Jiang* (dry Rhizoma Zingiberis), *Rou Gui* (Cortex Cinnamomi Cassiae), *Fu Zi* (Radix Lateralis Praeparatus Aconiti Carmichaeli), and the like. If what is precipitated is yellow and there is thirst, vexation and agitation, a vacuous pulse, and generalized fever, this is due to contained summerheat. One should, (therefore, use) *Huang Lian* (Rhizoma Coptidis Chinensis), *Bian Dou* (Semen Dolichoris Lablab), *Xiang Ru* (Herba Elsholtziae Seu Moslae), and the like. If what is precipitated is clear water or stale rotten matter which is the color of water and there is no abdominal pain but generalized heaviness, fatigue, lack of strength, and a deep, moderate pulse, this is due to dampness. One should, (therefore, use) *Cang Zhu* (Rhizoma Atractylodis), *Bai Zhu* (Rhizoma Atractylodis Macrocephalae), *Hou Po* (Cortex Magnolia Officinalis), and the like. If what is precipitated is untransformed grain of extraordinarily sour and stench-like smell and there is satiety and oppression in the chest and diaphragm and aversion to the smell of food, this is due to food damage. One should, (therefore, use) *Shan Zha* (Fructus Crataegi), *Cao Guo* (Fructus

Amomi Tsao-ko), *Shen Qu* (Massa Medica Fermentata), *Mai Ya* (Fructus Germinatus Hordei Vulgaris), *Lai Fu Zi* (Semen Raphani Sativi), and the like. If there is (sometimes) diarrhea and (sometimes) no diarrhea with the amounts of stools (sometimes) large and (sometimes) small or (the stool) is like fish gelatin, this is due to contained phlegm. One should, (therefore, use) *Nan Xing* (Rhizoma Arisaematis), *Ban Xia* (Rhizoma Pinelliae Ternatae), and the like. If precipitation is large in quantity and accompanied by inhibited urination, it is necessary to separate and disinhibit yin and yang to make voiding (of clear urine) long and the stools solid. This requires *Fu Ling* (Sclerotium Poriae Cocos), *Zhu Ling* (Sclerotium Polypori Umbellati), *Hua Shi* (Talcum), *Ze Xie* (Rhizoma Alismatis), and the like. These medicinals, however, cannot be prescribed in case of enduring diarrhea, for they will reduce yin qi. Otherwise the eyelids will be sunken, and the disease will become threatening. The above seven sections are concerned with evil-quelling medicinals.

As to spleen-fortifying medicinals, the best are *Bai Zhu* (Rhizoma Atractylodis Macrocephalae), *Fu Ling* (Sclerotium Poriae Cocos), *Chen Pi* (Pericarpium Citri Reticulatae), *Bai Shao* (Radix Albus Paeoniae Lactiflorae), and the like. Among those supplementing the spleen, the best are *Ren Shen* (Radix Panacis Ginseng), *Shan Yao* (Radix Paeoniae Lactiflorae), *Bian Dou* (Semen Dolichoris Lablab), *Lian Rou* (Semen Nelumbinis Nuciferae), *Yi Yi Ren* (Semen Coicis Lachryma-jobi), *Qian Shi* (Semen Euryalis Ferocis), and the like. Generally speaking, when the spleen and stomach qi ascends, the government of generation and growth works, and, when it descends, the government of gathering and storing works. In enduring diarrhea, the qi of the spleen and stomach is sunken below. This requires upbearing and effusing medicinals as assistants, such as *Sheng Ma* (Rhizoma Cimicifugae), *Fang Feng* (Radix Ledebouriellae Divaricatae), *Chai Hu* (Radix Bupleuri), *Ge Gen* (Radix Puerariae), and *Qiang Huo* (Radix Et Rhizoma Notopterygii). There is also diarrhea between the *zi* watch and the fifth watch.[48] This diarrhea is produced by kidney vacuity, requiring *Rou Kou* (Semen Myristicae Fragrantis), *Po Gu Zhi* (Fructus Psoraleae Corylifoliae), *Wu Zhu Yu*

---

[48] *I.e.*, from eleven p.m. to five a.m.

(Fructus Evodiae Rutecarpae), and *Wu Wei Zi* (Fructus Schisandrae Chinensis) to supplement the kidneys.

*Wu Ling San* (Poria Five [Ingredients] Powder) [See #3 above.]

*Wei Ling San* (Calm the Stomach Poria Powder)

To treat cold diarrhea with abdominal pain and uninhibited clear stools and urine, take one cupful of *Wei Ling San* which is decocted with *Jiang* (Rhizoma Zingiberis) and *Za Zao* (Fructus Zizyphi Jujubae) in water. [This is *Ping Wei San* {Calm the Stomach Powder} combined with *Wu Ling San* {Five (Ingredients) Poria Powder}.]

*Ru Ling Tang* (Elsholtzia & Poria Decoction)

Summerheat diarrhea with (the body) hot like boiling water, heart vexation, thirst and restlessness can be treated with *Ru Ling Tang*. It is composed of eight flavors. Decoct with one handful of *Deng Xin* (Medulla Junci Effusi). [This is *Huang Lian Xiang Ru Yin*, Coptis & Elsholtzia Beverage, combined with *Si Ling San*, Four (Ingredients) Poria Powder.]

*Chai Ling Tang* (Bupleurum & Poria Decoction)

(This treats) generalized fever and thirst in addition to frequent diarrhea. One dose of *Chai Ling Tang* can bring magically swift effect. [This is *Xiao Chai Hu Tang*, Minor Bupleurum Decoction, combined with *Wu Ling San*, Five (Ingredients) Poria Powder.]

*Shen Ling Bai Zhu San* (Ginseng, Poria & Atractylodes Powder)

(This formula is composed of) *Lian Rou* (Semen Nelumbinis Nuciferae), *Bian Dou* (Semen Dolichoris Lablab), *Yi Yi Ren* (Semen Coicis Lachryma-jobi), *Sha Ren* (Fructus Amomi), *Gan Cao* (Radix Glycyrrhizae), *Jie Geng* (Radix Platycodi Grandiflori), and *Shan Yao* (Radix Dioscoreae Oppositae). It treats enduring diarrhea with vacuity of the stomach.

# 19. Sudden Turmoil Is a Result of Spleen Cold & Food Damage

Sudden pain in the heart and abdomen with vomiting above and diarrhea below is called damp sudden turmoil. Gripping pain in the abdomen with desire but inability to vomit and desire but inability to evacuate is called dry sudden turmoil. This pathocondition is divided into the two species of cold and heat. In the cold species, that which is vomited and evacuated is a fishy, rotten (matter) which is a clear, cold liquid. The pulse is deep and slow and there is reversal cold of the limbs, abdominal pain, and no liking for water. This is due to overwhelming yin evils. In the hot species, there is vomiting and loose bowel movements, vexatious thirst, sweating, thirst with desire to drink cool water, a deep, rapid pulse, and warm limbs. This is due to overwhelming yang evils.

To treat any category (of sudden turmoil), use *Huo Xiang Zheng Qi San* (Agastaches Correct the Qi Powder) with additions and subtractions. For dry sudden turmoil, first apply mechanical ejection with brine and then administer *Huo Xiang Zheng Qi San* (Agastache Correct the Qi Powder) to regulate (the qi). If ejection cannot be provoked, death will come in no time.

*Huo Xiang Zheng Qi San* (Agastache Correct the Qi Powder)

*Zheng Qi San* is composed of *Ban Xia Qu* (Mass Medica Fermentata Cum Pinelliam), *Zi Su* (Folium Perillae Frutescentis), *Huo Xiang* (Herba Agastachis Seu Pogostemi), *Fu Ling* (Sclerotium Poriae Cocos), *Chen Pi* (Pericarpium Citri Reticulatae), *Bai Zhu* (Rhizoma Atractylodis Macrocephalae), *Bai Zhi* (Radix Angelicae Dahuricae), *Hou Po* (Cortex Magnoliae Officinalis), *Jie Geng* (Radix Platycodi Grandiflori), *Gan Cao* (Radix Glycyrrhizae), *Fu Pi* (Pericarpium Arecae Catechu), *Sheng Jiang* (uncooked Rhizoma Zingiberis), and *Da Zao* (Fructus Zizyphi Jujubae). It treats vomiting and diarrhea with contention between yin and yang. If there is heat, add ginger-fried *Huang Lian* (Rhizoma Coptidis Chinensis). If there is cold, add *Gan Jiang* (dry Rhizoma Zingiberis). For abdominal pain, add *Guan Gui* (tubiform Cortex Cinnamomi Cassiae). In case of severe abdominal pain, add *Wu Zhu Yu* (Fructus Evodiae Rutecarpae) and subtract *Huo Xiang* (Herba Agastachis Seu Pogostemi). For inhibited urination, add *Che Qian Zi* (Semen Plantaginis). For cramps, add *Mu Gua* (Fructus Chaenomelis Lagenariae). For fever and thirst, add *Mai Dong* (Tuber Ophiopogonis Japonici) and *Dan Zhu Ye* (Herba Lophatheri Gracilis). In case of frequently going to the latrine yet with inhibited defecation, add *Zhi Ke* (Fructus Citri Aurantii). In case of summerheat stroke, add *Bian Dou* (Semen Dolichoris Lablab) and *Xiang Ru* (Herba Elsholtziae Seu Moslae). For glomus below the heart, add *Zhi Shi* (Fructus Immaturus Citri Aurantii) and *Qing Pi* (Pericarpium Citri Reticulatae Viride). In case of inability to transform meat food, add *Shan Zha* (Fructus Crataegi). In case of inability to transform grain, add *Shen Qu* (Massa Medica Fermentata) and *Mai Ya* (Fructus Germinatus Hordei Vulgaris).

*Shao Yan Tang* (Burnt Salt Decoction)

Put a pinchful of salt on a knife and then burn (the knife) till red. Take the salt with child's urine or freshly drawn water. Presently ejection (*i.e.,* vomiting) will occur.

*Ji Jiu Hui Yang Tang* (Emergency Recover Yang Decoction)

(This is composed of) *Dang Shen* (Radix Codonopsitis Pilosulae), eight *qian*; *Fu Zi* (Radix Lateralis Praeparatus Aconiti Carmichaeli), eight *qian*; *Gan Jiang* (dry Rhizoma Zingiberis), four *qian*; *Bai Zhu* (Rhizoma Atractylodis Macrocephalae), four *qian*; *Gan Cao* (Radix Glycyrrhizae), three *qian*; *Tao Ren* (Semen Pruni Persicae), two *qian*; and *Hong Hua* (Flos Carthami Tinctorii), two *qian*. Decoct in water and administer.

# 20. Glomus Fullness Develops from Fatigued Spleen & Damp Accumulation

Glomus fullness is not the (same) glomus as in lump glomus, but (refers to) glomus oppression in the chest with discomfort and lack of smooth flow. Because the spleen is fatigued, it is not able to convey and transform water and grains. Therefore, dampness accumulates and develops into phlegm. This lodges in the central stomach duct, producing a feeling of glomus oppression. The appropriate treatment is to fortify the spleen and normalize the flow of qi. Once the qi is normalized, phlegm is disinhibited. When the spleen is fortified, food is transformed. Then glomus is dispersed, and free flow and health are regained.

The formula to use (for this) is *Er Chen Tang* (Two Aged [Ingredients] Decoction) plus *Zhi Shi* (Fructus Immaturus Citri Aurantii), *Bai Zhu* (Rhizoma Atractylodis Macrocephalae), *Xiang Fu* (Rhizoma Cyperi Rotundi), *Sha Ren* (Fructus Amomi), *Bai Dou Kou* (Fructus Cardamomi), *Huo Xiang* (Herba Agastachis Seu Pogostemi), *Hou Po* (Cortex Magnolia Officinalis), etc. Thin persons are liable to have depressed heat. (For them,) add *Huang Lian* (Rhizoma Coptidis Chinensis) and subtract *Ban Xia* (Rhizoma Pinelliae Ternatae). (In case of) blood vacuity, add *Chuan Xiong* (Radix Ligustici Wallichii) and *Dang Gui* (Radix Angelicae Sinensis) and subtract *Ban Xia* (Rhizoma Pinelliae Ternatae). (In case of) food accumulation, add *Shen Qu* (Massa Medica Fermentata), *Mai Ya* (Fructus Germinatus Hordei Vulgaris) and *Shan Zha* (Fructus Crataegi) and subtract *Bai Zhu* (Rhizoma Atractylodis Macrocephalae) and *Ban Xia* (Rhizoma Pinelliae Ternatae). Fat persons are liable to have damp phlegm. (For them,) add *Cang Zhu* (Rhizoma Atractylodis). (In case of) qi vacuity, add *Ren Shen* (Radix Panacis Ginseng) and subtract *Ban Xia* (Rhizoma Pinelliae Ternatae). (In case of) phlegm obstruction, add *Gua Lou* (Fructus Trichosanthis Kirlowii), *Bei Mu* (Bulbus Fritillariae), *Jie Geng* (Radix Platycodi Grandiflori), *Zhu Li* (Succus Bambusae), and *Jiang Zhi* (Succus Rhizomatis Zingiberis) and remove *Bai Zhu* (Rhizoma Atractylodis Macrocephalae) and *Ban Xia* (Rhizoma Pinelliae Ternatae). (In case of) spleen dampness with fullness of the center, add *Cang Zhu* (Rhizoma Atractylodis) and *Shao Yao* (Radix Paeoniae Lactiflorae) and remove *Ban Xia* (Rhizoma Pinelliae Ternatae).

*Er Chen Tang* (Two Aged [Ingredients] Decoction) [See chapter 11 above.]

# 21. Hiccup Is Due to Stomach Qi Not Flowing Normally

Hiccup is popularly known as breath-catching. If the noise is short, it comes from the middle burner. This is a disease of water and grains. If the noise is long, it comes from the lower burner. This is due to vacuity and evils mutually contending. If the pulse is floating and moderate, this is favorable. If it is bowstring and tense, this is dangerous.

If hiccup is due to constipation caused by the mistake of not treating cold damage with precipitation, then use *Cheng Qi Tang* (Order the Qi Decoction). For hiccup due to stomach cold as the sequela of vomiting and diarrhea, use *Ding Xiang Shi Di Tang* (Clove & Persimmon Calyx Decoction). For hiccup due to stomach heat as the sequela of vomiting and diarrhea, use *Ju Pi Zhu Ru Tang* (Orange Peel & Bamboo Shavings Decoction). For qi coun-terflow hiccup, use *Mu Xiang Tiao Qi San* (Auklandia Regulate the Qi Powder). Hiccup following a disease is difficult to treat.

*Cheng Qi Tang* (Order the Qi Decoction) [See #3 above.]

*Ding Xiang Shi Di Tang* (Clove & Persimmon Calyx Decoction)

*Ding Xiang Shi Di Tang* is a decoction including *Ren Shen* (Radix Panacis Ginseng) and *Sheng Jiang* (uncooked Rhizoma Zingiberis). Taking it quiets stomach cold (hiccup) after vomiting and diarrhea (or) cold damage.

*Ju Pi Zhu Ru Tang* (Orange Peel & Bamboo Shavings Decoction)

*Ju Pi Zhu Ru Tang* is a decoction including *Ren Shen* (Radix Panacis Ginseng), *Gan Cao* (Radix Glycyrrhizae), *Sheng Jiang* (uncooked Rhizoma Zingiberis) and *Da Zao* (Fructus Zizyphi Jujubae). Taking it quiets stomach heat (hiccup).

*Mu Xiang Tiao Qi San* (Auklandia Regulate the Qi Powder)

*Mu Xiang Tiao Qi San* includes *Ding Xiang* (Flos Caryophylli), *Bai Kou Ren* (Fructus Cardamomi), *Huo Xiang* (Herba Agastachis Seu Pogostemi), *Tan Xiang* (Lignum Santali Albi), *Sha Ren* (Fructus Amomi), and *Gan Cao* (Radix Glycyrrhizae).

## 22. Cough Is Due to the Lung Qi Not Clearing

Jie-gu[49] said:

> Cough may be without phlegm but with noise. This is due to damaged lung qi not clearing. Cough may be without noise but with phlegm. The phlegm is produced by the spleen which is affected by dampness. Cough may be with (both) phlegm and noise. This is due to damaged lung qi stirring and spleen dampness.

Dan-xi categorized cough as wind cold, phlegm-rheum, fire depression, taxation coughing, and lung distention. According to the annotation made by Dai Yuan-li, (the complications of) nasal congestion, heavy voice, and aversion to cold reveal wind cold. If phlegm noise is heard when coughing and coughing terminates when phlegm is coughed up, these are indications of phlegm rheum. Noise (of phlegm), scanty phlegm, and a red facial complexion are indications of fire depression. Night sweats, copious phlegm, and (alternating) cold and heat are (characteristic of) taxation cough. Panting and fullness arising on movement with rapid breathing and heavy breathing reveal lung distention.

In relation to cough, if the pulse is floating and tight, there is vacuity cold. If it is deep and rapid, there is repletion heat. If it is surging and slippery, there is abundant phlegm. If it is bowstring and choppy, there is shortage of blood. If it is floating and large, this is favorable. If it is deep and small, this is dangerous.

For wind cold coughing, use *Su Chen Jiu Bao Yin* (Perilla & Aquilaria Nine Treasures Drink). For phlegm rheum cough, use *Dao Tan Tang* (Abduct

---

[49] A.k.a. Zhang Yuan-su

Phlegm Decoction). If (cough) is very severe, use *Xiao Wei Dan* (Minor Stomach Elixir). For fire depression coughing, use *Shen Su Yin* (Ginseng & Perilla Drink) removing *Ren Shen* (Radix Panacis Ginseng) and adding *Ku Qin* (old Radix Scutellariae Baicalensis). For taxation coughing, use *Zhi Mu Fu Ling Tang* (Anemarrhena & Poria Decoction) or *Qing Li Zi Kan Tang* (Clear Fire & Enrich Water Decoction). For enduring cough, use *Kuan Dong Hua* (Flos Tussilaginis Farfarae), *Zi Wan* (Radix Asteris Tatarici), *Wu Wei Zi* (Fructus Schisandrae Chinensis), and *Wu Mei Rou* (Fructus Pruni Mume), all in equal amounts. Make into pills and melt in the mouth. For lung distention cough, use *Qing Fei Yin* (Clear the Lungs Drink).

*Su Chen Jiu Bao Yin* (Perilla & Aquilaria Nine Treasures Drink)

*Su Chen Jiu Bao Yin* includes *Ma Huang* (Herba Ephedrae), *Rou Gui* (Cortex Cinnamomi Cassiae), *Bo He* (Herba Menthae Haplocalysis), *Chen Pi* (Pericarpium Citri Reticulatae), *Xing Ren* (Semen Pruni Armeniacae), *Gan Cao* (Radix Glycyrrhizae), and *Da Fu Pi* (Pericarpium Arecae Catechu). It is miraculously effective for cold cough.

*Dao Tan Tang* (Abduct Phlegm Decoction) [See chapter 11.]

*Xiao Wei Dan* (Minor Stomach Elixir)

*Xiao Wei Dan* uses vinegar-processed *Yuan Hua* (Flos Daphnes Genkwae), *Da Ji* (Herba Seu Radix Cirsii Japonici), *Gan Sui* (Radix Euphorbiae Kansui), *Da Huang* (Radix Et Rhizoma Rhei), and *Huang Bai* (Cortex Phellodendri). Boil *Bai Zhu* (Rhizoma Atractylodis Macrocephalae) down to a paste and mix (with the above medicinals), making them into pills. Take with hot water on an empty stomach before going to sleep.

*Shen Su Yin* (Ginseng & Perilla Drink) [See #6 above.]

*Zhi Mu Fu Ling Tang* (Anemarrhena & Poria Decoction)

*Zhi Mu Fu Ling Tang* includes *Dang Gui* (Radix Angelicae Sinensis), *Bai Shao* (Radix Albus Paeoniae Lactiflorae), *Di Huang* (Radix Rehmanniae), *Tian Dong* (Tuber Asparagi Cochinensis), *Gan Cao* (Radix Glycyrrhizae), and *Bai Zhu* (Rhizoma Atractylodis Macrocephalae). It is a good formula for taxation coughing.

*Qing Fei Yin* (Clear the Lungs Drink)

*Qing Fei Yin* is composed of *Zhi Zi* (Fructus Gardeniae Jasminoidis), *Huang Qin* (Radix Scutellariae Baicalensis), *Sang Pi* (Cortex Radicis Mori Albi), *Dang Gui* (Radix Angelicae Sinensis), *Fu Ling* (Sclerotium Poriae Cocos), *Tian Dong* (Tuber Asparagi Cochinensis), *Mai Dong* (Tuber Ophiopogonis Japonici), *Jie Geng* (Radix Platycodi Grandiflori), *Chen Pi* (Pericarpium Citri Reticulatae), *Gan Cao* (Radix Glycyrrhizae), *Xing Ren* (Semen Pruni Armeniacae), *Wu Wei Zi* (Fructus Schisandrae Chinensis), *Sheng Jiang* (uncooked Rhizoma Zingiberis), and *Da Zao* (Fructus Zizyphi Jujubae). Decoct in water and administer.

*Qing Li Zi Kan Tang* (Clear Li [*i.e.*, Fire] & Enrich Kan [*i.e.*, Water] Decoction)

This is for taxation coughing. It is composed of *Dan Pi* (Cortex Radicis Moutan), *Bai Zhu* (Rhizoma Atractylodis Macrocephalae), *Ze Xie* (Rhizoma Alismatis), *Bai Shao* (Radix Albus Paeoniae Lactiflorae), *Yu Rou* (Fructus Corni Officinalis), *Shan Yao* (Radix Dioscoreae Oppositae), *Gan Cao* (Radix Glycyrrhizae), *Fu Ling* (Sclerotium Poriae Cocos), *Tian Dong* (Tuber Asparagi Cochinensis), *Mai Dong* (Tuber Ophiopogonis Japonici), *Dang Gui* (Radix Angelicae Sinensis), *Sheng Di* (uncooked Radix Rehmanniae), *Shu Di* (cooked Radix Rehmanniae), *Zhi Mu* (Rhizoma Anemarrhenae Asphodeloidis), and *Huang Bai* (Cortex Phellodendri). It clears *kan* and *li*.[50]

# 23. Eructation Is Invariably
# Impugned to Phlegm (or) Fire

If eructation is due to phlegm and fire in the stomach, use *Nan Xing* (Rhizoma Arisaematis), *Ban Xia* (Rhizoma Pinelliae Ternatae), *Shi Gao*

---

[50] *Kan* and *li* are two trigrams respectively representing fire/south/heart and water/north/kidneys.

(Gypsum Fibrosum), *Xiang Fu* (Rhizoma Cyperi Rotundi), and stir-fried *Shan Zhi* (Fructus Gardeniae Jasminoidis). Either pills or decoction is alright. For cold stomach eructation, use *Er Chen Tang* (Two Aged [Ingredients] Decoction) plus *Gan Jiang* (dry Rhizoma Zingiberis), *Yi Zhi* (Fructus Alpiniae Oxyphyllae), and *Mu Xiang* (Radix Auklandiae Lappae). Some women may suffer from eructation. They must belch more than 10 times before coming to an end. After the belching, they will feel relief of the heart, but if they fail to belch, they will feel tight and oppressed (in the chest). (In that case,) the use of *Yue Ju Wan* (Out-thrust Tribulation Pills) is effective.

## 24. Swallowing Acid Is, Without Exception, the Work of Food Collection

Swallowing acid is acid water pricking the heart. Acid vomiting is vomiting of acid water. Both cases are ascribed to spleen vacuity which is unable to convey and transform drink and food. (If these) become depressed and accumulate for a long time, heat is generated from dampness. Damp heat (then) steams so as to produce acidity. This requires *Ping Wei San* (Calm the Stomach Powder) plus *Shen Qu* (Massa Medica Fermentata), *Mai Ya* (Fructus Germinatus Hordei Vulgaris), carbonized *Shan Zha* (Fructus Crataegi), *Cao Guo* (Fructus Amomi Tsao-ko), *Wu Zhu Yu* (Fructus Evodiae Rutecarpae), *Huang Lian* (Rhizoma Coptidis Chinensis), and *Zhi Shi* (Fructus Immaturus Citri Aurantii). The use of *Liu Yu Tang* (Six Depressions Decoction) or *Yue Ju Wan* (Out-thrust Tribulation Pills) is even more wonderful. For vomiting of clear water, use *Cang Zhu* (Rhizoma Atractylodis), *Bai Zhu* (Rhizoma Atractylodis Macrocephalae), *Chen Pi* (Pericarpium Citri Reticulatae), *Fu Ling* (Sclerotium Poriae Cocos), and *Hua Shi* (Talcum), all in equal amounts. Decocted in water and administered, this is effective.

## Appendix: Clamoring Stomach Pathocondition

Clamoring stomach is popularly called clamoring heart. It may be caused by phlegm stirred up by fire. This requires *Er Chen Tang* (Two Aged

[Ingredients] Decoction) plus wine stir-fried *Huang Lian* (Rhizoma Coptidis Chinensis), and *Zhi Zi Ren* (Fructus Gardeniae Jasminoidis). It (also) may be caused by shortage of heart blood. This requires *Ba Zhen Tang* (Eight Pearls Decoction) plus *Mai Dong* (Tuber Ophiopogonis Japonici), *Zhi Zi* (Fructus Gardeniae Jasminoidis), *Chen Pi* (Pericarpium Citri Reticulatae), *Wu Mei* (Fructus Pruni Mume), and stir-fried *Mi* (Semen Oryzae Sativae). Or it may be caused by food depression. To treat this, use *Yue Ju Wan* (Out-thrust Tribulation Pills).

*Ping Wei San* (Calm the Stomach Powder) [See chapter 13.]

*Liu Yu Tang* (Six Depressions Decoction) [See #14 above.]

*Yue Ju Wan* (Out-thrust Tribulation Pills) [See #14 above.]

*Er Chen Tang* (Two Aged [Ingredients] Decoction) [See chapter 11.]

*Ba Zhen Tang* (Eight Pearls Decoction) [See chapter 10.]

# 25. Center Fullness Drum Distention Is Due to Vacuous Spleen Not Moving

If there is center fullness drum distention without swelling of the four limbs, this is simply abdominal distention. It looks like a drum and is, therefore, called drum distention. According to the *Ren Zhai Zhi Zhi (The Direct Guide [Composed in] the Benevolence Study)*[51], this pathocondition is divided into four categories: qi drum, blood drum, food drum, and water drum distention. All these categories are due to the spleen being too vacuous to move and transform water and grains. In consequence, (water and grains) collect and gather so as to give rise to distention. The appropriate treat-ments are to normalize the qi, harmonize the blood, loosen the center, and disinhibit water. Each (of these treatments) has its own indications. By no means should one use drastic medicinals which

---

[51] The *Ren Zhai Zhi Zhi Fang Lun* (*Treatise on Formulary, A Direct Guide to the Benevolent Study*) in full, a medical work by Yang Ren-ying of the Southern Song dynasty.

might result in damaging the spleen and stomach. If the umbilicus protrudes and the belly is enlarged with bulging greenish blue veins or if the insteps of the feet and the palms become flat, this is usually difficult to treat.

Drum distention in women may be caused by qi (or) food, but, in most cases, it develops from the blood division. If distention is produced by qi (or) food, the abdomen is distended but there is no menstrual block. If it is produced by the blood division, there is invariably menstrual block (i.e., amenorrhea).

In relation to distention and fullness, if the pulse is bowstring, the spleen is restrained by the liver. If it is surging and rapid, there is heat. If it is slow and weak, there is vacuity cold. If it is floating, there is vacuity fullness. If it is tight, there is repletion in the ce nter. If it is floating and large, (the condition) is curable. If it is vacuous and small, (the condition) is dangerous and critical. Loosening (i.e., relief) in the morning and tightening (i.e., exacerbation) in the evening reveal blood vacuity. Loosening in the evening and tightening in the morning reveal qi vacuity. Tightness in both the morning and evening shows vacuity of both the qi and blood.

To treat abdominal distention in fat persons, I use Wei Ling Tang (Stomach Poria Decoction). For abdominal distention in thin persons, (I) use Ru Ling Tang (Elsholtzia & Poria Decoction). Both formulas bring rapid effect.

Fen Xiao Tang (Separating & Dispersing Decoction)

Fen Xiao Tang treats drum distention. It is composed of Cang Zhu (Rhizoma Atractylodis), Bai Zhu (Rhizoma Atractylodis Macrocephalae), Chen Pi (Pericarpium Citri Reticulatae), Xiang Fu (Rhizoma Cyperi Rotundi), Hou Po (Cortex Magnoliae Officinalis), Zhi Shi (Fructus Immaturus Citri Aurantii), Fu Ling (Sclerotium Poriae Cocos), Mu Xiang (Radix Auklandiae Lappae), and Sha Ren (Fructus Amomi) with Fu Pi (Pericarpium Arecae Catechu), Zhu Ling (Sclerotium Polypori Umbellati), and Ze Xie (Rhizoma Alismatis) as assistants. Decoct in water with three pieces of Sheng Jiang (uncooked Rhizoma Zingiberis) and a handful of

*Deng Xin* (Medulla Junci Effusi), and administer. In case of rapid breathing, add *Chen Xiang* (Lignum Aquilariae Agallochae). If there is rib-side pain with a black facial complexion, this is qi drum distention. (In this case,) add *Qing Pi* (Pericarpium Citri Reticulatae Viride) and remove *Bai Zhu* (Rhizoma Atractylodis Macrocephalae). If there is rib-side fullness and lower abdominal distention and pain with blood threads (visible) in the body, this is blood drum distention. (In that case,) add *Dang Gui* (Radix Angelicae Sinensis), *Chi Shao* (Radix Rubrus Paeoniae Lactiflorae), *Hong Hua* (Flos Carthami Tinctorii), and *Dan Pi* (Cortex Radicis Moutan) and remove *Bai Zhu* (Rhizoma Atractylodis Macrocephalae) and *Fu Ling* (Sclerotium Poriae Cocos). Abdominal distention with eructation, acid regurgitation, (persistent) satiety, and oppression is food drum distention. (For such a case,) add *Shan Zha* (Fructus Crataegi), *Shen Qu* (Massa Medica Fermentata), *Mai Ya* (Fructus Germinatus Hordei Vulgaris), and *Lai Fu Zi* (Semen Raphani Sativi) and remove *Bai Zhu* (Rhizoma Atractylodis Macrocephalae) and *Fu Ling* (Sclerotium Poriae Cocos). If there is aversion to cold, reversal cold of the hands and feet, and diarrhea with clear water, this is water drum distention. Add *Gui Zhi* (Ramulus Cinnamomi Cassiae). Drum-like distention and fullness of the chest and abdomen with lumps is drum distention developing from dispersed glomus. (For this,) add *Shan Zha* (Fructus Crataegi), *Shen Qu* (Massa Medica Fermentata), *Mai Ya* (Fructus Germinatus Hordei Vulgaris), *Ban Xia* (Rhizoma Pinelliae Ternatae), *Qing Pi* (Pericarpium Citri Reticulatae Viride), *Gui Wei* (Apex Radicis Angelicae Sinensis), *Yuan Hu Suo* (Rhizoma Corydalis Yanhusuo), and *Bie Jia* (Carapax Amydae Sinensis) and remove *Bai Zhu* (Rhizoma Atractylodis Macrocephalae), *Fu Ling* (Sclerotium Poriae Cocos), *Zhu Ling* (Sclerotium Polypori Umbellati), and *Ze Xie* (Rhizoma Alismatis).

*Wei Ling Tang* (Calm the Stomach Poria Decoction) and *Ru Ling Tang* (Elsholtza & Poria Decoction) [See #18 above.]

# Appendix: Puffy Swelling

The *Nei Jing (Inner Classic)* says:

> All dampness with swelling and fullness are ascribed to the spleen. All qi rushing and depression are ascribed to the lungs.

The cause of vacuity swelling is invariably vacuity of the spleen failing to move and depressed and blocked lungs. In consequence, water soaks through the triple burner, producing puffy swelling. (The skin) becomes pitted when pressed but gradually becomes level (again) after pressure is relieved. If there is generalized fever, water qi is located in the exterior and its treatment should be sweating. If there is no generalized fever, water qi is located in the interior, and its treatment should be precipitation. It also states that swelling above the lumbus necessitates sweating, while swelling below the lumbus necessitates disinhibition of urination. At the same time, if it is a good method, it should also normalize the qi and harmonize the spleen. One should be careful not to use drastically (precipitating) medicinals like *Da Ji* (Herba Seu Radix Cirsii Japonici), *Yuan Hua* (Flos Daphnes Genkwae), and *Gan Sui* (Radix Euphorbiae Kansui) to attack a vacuity pathocondition. I fear that it is easy to break (the dam) but it is difficult to secure and stop it up (again). Once water comes back, there will be no mechanism (*i.e.*, no way) to treat it.

Wind swelling is characterized by numbness and migratory pain in the skin. To treat it, use *Fen Xin Qi Yin* (Separate the Heart Qi Drink). Qi swelling is characterized by emaciated limbs and distention and fullness of the chest and rib-side. To treat it, use *Liu Qi Yin* (Qi Flow Drink) with additions and subtractions. In respect to water swelling, swelling above the lumbus should be treated with *Fen Xin Qi Yin* (Separate the Heart Qi Drink), while swelling below the lumbus should be treated with *Wu Zi Shi Pi Yin* (Five Seeds & Ten Peels Drink). Blood swelling is characterized by red blood threads in the skin. Women are liable to have this pattern. It is due to vanquished blood transforming into water. *Tiao Jing San* (Regulate Menses Powder) can treat it. For swelling produced by sores, take *Bai Du San* (Vanquish Toxins Powder) plus *Jing Jie* (Herba Schizonepetae

Tenuifoliae), *Fang Feng* (Radix Ledebouriellae Divaricatae), and *Jin Yin Hua* (Flos Lonicerae Japonicae), occasionally administering *Wu Zi Shi Pi Yin* (Five Seeds & Ten Peels Beverage) instead. Swollen insteps due to spleen vacuity following a disease are caused by the center qi sunken below. This requires *Bu Zhong Yi Qi Tang* (Supplement the Center & Boost the Qi Decoction). For swelling due to failure to acclimatize to water and earth (*i.e.*, a new environment) in a strange place, use *Huo Xiang Zheng Qi San* (Agastache Correct the Qi Powder). When swelling has basically abated, it is appropriate to use a paste made from boiled-down *Bai Zhu* (Rhizoma Atractylodis Macrocephalae) to regulate the spleen and stomach.

*Fen Xin Qi Yin* (Separate the Heart Qi Drink)

*Fen Xin Qi* includes *Er Chen Tang* (Two Aged [Ingredients] Decoction) plus *Mu Tong* (Caulis Akebiae), *Guan Gui* (tubiform Cortex Cinnamomi Cassiae), *Fu Pi* (Pericarpium Arecae Catechu), *Qing Pi* (Pericarpium Citri Reticulatae Viride), *San Pi* (Cortex Radicis Mori Albi), *Su Geng* (Caulis Perillae Frutescentis), *Qiang Huo* (Radix Et Rhizoma Notopterygii), *Shao Yao* (Radix Paeoniae Lactiflorae), *Sheng Jiang* (uncooked Rhizoma Zingiberis), *Da Zao* (Fructus Zizyphi Jujubae), and *Deng Xin* (Medulla Junci Effusi).

*Liu Qi Yin* (Qi Flow Drink)

*Liu Qi Yin* is composed of *Mu Xiang* (Radix Auklandiae Lappae), *Zi Su* (Folium Perillae Frutescentis), *Chen Pi* (Pericarpium Citri Reticulatae), *Fu Ling* (Sclerotium Poriae Cocos), *Ban Xia* (Rhizoma Pinelliae Ternatae), *Hou Po* (Cortex Magnoliae Officinalis), *Bai Zhu* (Rhizoma Atractylodis Macrocephalae), *Fu Pi* (Pericarpium Arecae Catechu), *Bing Lang* (Semen Arecae Catechu), *Mu Gua* (Fructus Chaenomelis Lagenariae), *Zhi Ke* (Fructus Citri Aurantii), *E Zhu* (Rhizoma Curcumae Zedoariae), *Bai Zhi* (Radix Angelicae Dahuricae), *Rou Gui* (Cortex Cinnamomi Cassiae), *Huo Xiang* (Herba Agastachis Seu Pogostemi), and *Chang Pu* (Rhizoma Acori Graminei).

*Wu Zi Shi Pi Yin* (Five Seeds & Ten Peels Drink)[52]

*Wu Zi Shi Pi Yin* is composed of *Che Qian Zi* (Semen Plantaginis), *Ting Li Zi* (Semen Lepidii Seu Descurainiae), *Zi Su Zi* (Fructus Perillae Frutescentis), *Ding Xiang Zi* (Semen Caryo-phylli), *Wu Jia Pi* (Cortex Radicis Acanthopanacis), *Sang Pi* (Cortex Radicis Mori Albi), *Fu Ling Pi* (Cortex Sclerotii Poriae Cocos), *Da Fu Pi* (Peri-carpium Arecae Catechu), *Ju Pi* (Pericarpium Citri Reticulatae), *Mu Gua Pi* (Pericarpium Fructi Chaeno-melis Lagenariae), *Mi* (Semen Oryzae Sativae), *Mu Tong Pi* (Pericarpium Akebiae), *Qing Pi* (Pericarpium Citri Reticulatae Viride), and *Jiang Pi* (Cortex Rhizomatis Zingiberis).

*Tiao Jing San* (Regulate Menses Powder)

*Tiao Jing* is composed of *Dang Gui* (Radix Angelicae Sinensis), *Yi Mu* (Herba Leonuri Heterophylli), *Sheng Di* (uncooked Radix Rehmanniae), *Dan Shen* (Radix Salviae Miltiorrhizae), *Niu Xi* (Radix Achyranthis Bidentatae), *Dan Pi* (Cortex Radicis Moutan), *Yuan Hu Suo* (Rhizoma Corydalis Yanhusuo), and a small amount of *Hong Hua* (Flos Carthami Tinctorii).

*Bai Du San* (Vanquish Toxins Powder) [See #4 above.]

*Bu Zhong Yi Qi Tang* (Supplement the Center & Boost the Qi Decoction) [See #5 above.]

*Huo Xiang Zheng Qi San* (Agastache Correct the Qi Powder) [See #19 above.]

---

[52] Since there are less than ten "peels" in this formula, another formula with a similar name is given here for reference. It is composed of *Fu Ling Pi* (Cortex Sclerotii Poriae Cocos), *Dan Pi* (Cortex Radicis Moutan), *Wu Jia Pi* (Cortex Radicis Acanthopanacis), *Gan Cao Pi* (Cortex Radicis Glycyrrhizae), *Mu Tong Pi* (Pericarpium Akebiae), *Cao Guo Pi* (Pericarpium Fructi Amomi Tsao-ko), *Di Gu Pi* (Cortex Radicis Lycii Chinensis), *Da Fu Pi* (Pericarpium Arecae Catechu), *Mu Gua Pi* (Pericarpium Fructi Lagenariae), *Sheng Jiang Pi* (Cortex Rhizomatis Zingiberis), *Tu Si Zi* (Semen Cuscutae Chinensis), *Che Qian Zi* (Semen Plantaginis), *Zi Su Zi* (Fructus Perillae Frutescentis), *Ting Li Zi* (Semen Lepidii Seu Descurainiae), and *Da Fu Zi* (Semen Arecae Catechu).

## 26. Dysphagia Occlusion & Stomach Reflux Are Due to Qi & Food Congealed Together

The disease of dysphagia occlusion is due to damage by excesses of the seven affects and dietary lack of discipline. Because of qi counterflow, food is unable to descend, and because of food obstruction, the qi is unable to move. (As a result,) qi, food, and phlegm congeal and bind together. If they lodge in the esophagus, dysphagia arises. If they lodge in the chest around the diaphragm, occlusion arises. They are in the way of drink and food, gradually giving rise to retching and vomiting which is the disease of stomach reflux.

Dan-xi said:

> Accumulation develops from the qi, and phlegm develops from accumulation. When phlegm contains static blood, it produces lumps.

If this pathocondition is not treated early enough, it is bound to become a difficult disease. In its initial stage, use *Wu Ge Kuan Zhong San* (Five Occlusions Loosen the Center Powder). If it endures for (many) days, use *Er Chen Tang* (Two Aged [Ingredients] Decoction) with additions and subtractions.

For both dysphagia occlusion and stomach reflux, use *Er Chen Tang* (Two Aged [Ingredients] Decoction) plus *Jiang Zhi* (Succus Rhizomatis Zingiberis) and *Zhu Li* (Succus Bambusae) as the ruling (prescription). For white (*i.e.*, pale complexioned), fat persons with qi vacuity, add *Ren Shen* (Radix Panacis Ginseng) and *Bai Zhu* (Rhizoma Atractylodis Macrocephalae). For thin, weak persons with blood vacuity, add *Dang Gui* (Radix Angelicae Sinensis), *Shao Yao* (Radix Paeoniae Lactiflorae), *Tao Ren* (Semen Pruni Persicae), and *Hong Hua* (Flos Carthami Tinctorii). If there is heat and oppression in the chest, add earthstir-fried *Huang Qin* (Radix Scutellariae Baicalensis), *Huang Lian* (Rhizoma Coptidis Chinensis), *Gua Lou* (Fructus Trichosanthis Kirlowii), and *Jie Geng* (Radix Platycodi Grandiflori) and remove *Ban Xia* (Rhizoma Pinelliae Ternatae). If the cause is binding depression of the seven affects, add *Xiang Fu* (Rhizoma Cyperi Rotundi), *Chuan Xiong* (Radix Ligustici Wallichii), *Mu Xiang* (Radix

126

Auklandiae Lappae), *Bing Lang* (Semen Arecae Catechu), and *Sha Ren* (Fructus Amomi). In case of spleen vacuity with failure to convey and transform, add *Ren Shen* (Radix Panacis Ginseng), *Shen Qu* (Massa Medica Fermentata) and *Mai Ya* (Fructus Germinatus Hordei Vulgaris) to assist (the spleen). If the stool is dry and bound, add a small amount of wine-steamed *Da Huang* (Radix Et Rhizoma Rhei) and mashed *Tao Ren* (Semen Pruni Persicae) to moisten it. Generally, in dysphagia occlusion disease, the blood is desiccated and the stomach duct is dry. (Therefore, patients) have difficulty taking pills. It is appropriate to boil down (the medicinals) to a paste and administer (this).

*Wu Ge Kuan Zhong San* (Five Occlusions Loosen the Center Powder)

*Wu Ge Kuan Zhong San* is composed of *Qing Pi* (Pericarpium Citri Reticulatae Viride), *Chen Pi* (Pericarpium Citri Reticulatae), *Ding Xiang* (Flos Caryophylli), *Mu Xiang* (Radix Auklandiae Lappae), *Bai Dou Kou* (Fructus Cardamomi), *Sha Ren* (Fructus Amomi), *Xiang Fu* (Rhizoma Cyperi Rotundi), *Hou Po* (Cortex Magnoliae Officinalis), *Gan Cao* (Radix Glycyrrhizae), *Yan* (Salt), and *Jiang* (Rhizoma Zingiberis).

*Er Chen Tang* (Two Aged [Ingredients] Decoction) [See chapter 11.]

# 27. Rapid Panting Has Vacuity & Has Repletion (Types)

Panting in a sudden disease is classified as repletion, and panting in an enduring disease is classified as vacuity. If the pulse is slippery and the four limbs are warm, it is easy to treat. If the pulse is choppy and the four limbs are·cold, it is difficult to medicate (*i.e.*, treat). If phlegm noise is heard once there is panting, this is due to phlegm. Panting now advancing and now subsiding, getting better on eating but returning after finishing eating is due to fire. Qi arising from below the umbilicus and surging straight up into the clear path (*i.e.*, the windpipe) reveals yin vacuity. Short, rapid breathing with no phlegm noise indicates qi vacuity. Panting with aversion to cold, fever, and a floating, tight pulse is due to wind cold. Panting with a gurgling noise, fearful (throbbing), and palpitations are due to water collecting below the heart. Generally speaking, when a disease has advanced to such (a stage) as to occasion panting, it is already a malign (*i.e.*, mortal) pathocondition. It is anything but easy to treat.

To treat panting, the (empirically) proven prescription is using *Su Zi Jiang Qi Tang* (Perilla Fruit Downbear Qi Decoction) as the ruling formula. For phlegm panting, add *Zhu Li* (Succus Bambusae). For fire panting, add *Zhi Zi* (Fructus Gardeniae Jasminoidis) and *Ku Qin* (old Radix Scutellariae Baicalensis). In case of yin vacuity, add *Zhi Mu* (Rhizoma Anemarrhenae Asphodeloidis), *Huang Bai* (Cortex Phellodendri), and *Zhu Li* (Succus Bambusae). In case of qi vacuity, add *Ren Shen* (Radix Panacis Ginseng) and *E Jiao* (Gelatinum Corii Asini). In case of wind cold, add *Su Ye* (Folium Perillae Frutescentis), *Ma Huang* (Herba Ephedrae), and *Xing Ren* (Semen Pruni Armeniacae).

(To treat) water panting, bake and then grind *Jiao Mu* (Semen Zanthoxyli Bungeani) and take with a decoction of two *qian* of *Sheng Jiang* (uncooked Rhizoma Zingiberis). In case of phlegm fire panting and coughing, regularly taking *Yu Lu Shuang* (Jade Dew Frost)[53] may eradicate the root of the disease.

*Su Zi Jiang Qi Tang* (Perilla Fruit Downbear Qi Decoction)

*Su Zi Jiang Qi Tang* includes *Er Chen Tang* (Two Aged [Ingredients] Decoction) plus *Jie Geng* (Radix Platycodi Grandiflori), *Wu Wei Zi* (Fructus Schisandrae Chinensis), *Sang Pi* (Cortex Radicis Mori Albi), *Gua Lou* (Fructus Trichosanthis Kirlowii), and *Zhi Ke* (Fructus Citri Aurantii). It can relieve panting and coughing instantly.

# 28. Tetany Has Yin & Yang (Types)

Tetany is contraction and hypertonicity of the nape of the neck and arched rigidity of the upper and lower back. (The patient) looks like a bird

---

[53] This refers to a white-skinned variety of litchi produced in Xinhui county, Guangdong Province.

with wings extended. Therefore, this is called tugging tetany. If it is caused by cold, the (sick) person suffers from absence of sweating and aversion to cold. This is called hard tetany and is categorized as yang. If it is caused by dampness, the (sick) person sweats but is not averse to cold. This is called soft tetany and is categorized as yin.

For either of these, use *Xiao Xu Ming Tang* (Minor Prolong Destiny [*i.e.,* Life] Decoction). If there is sweating, remove *Ma Huang* (Herba Ephedrae). If diaphoresis is overdone or too much blood is lost, there will be no blood (left) to nourish the sinews. As a result, the sinews become tense and contracted, and the hundreds of joints become rigid. For such tetany, use *Shi Quan Da Bu Tang* (Ten [Ingredients] Completely & Greatly Supplementing Decoction).

*Xiao Xu Ming Tang* (Minor Prolong Destiny Decoction) [See #7 above.]

*Shi Quan Da Bu Tang* (Ten [Ingredients] Completely & Greatly Supplementing Decoction) [See chapter 9.]

# 29. The Five Accumulations & Six Gatherings Are Nothing Other Than Qi Congealed with Phlegm & Blood

The five viscera are subject to accumulation, and the six bowels to gathering. Accumulation is categorized as yin and occurs in a fixed place. Gathering is categorized as yang and has no constant shape. Accumulation of the liver is called fat qi.[54] Accumulation of the heart is called hidden beam.[55] Accumulation of the spleen is called glomus qi.[56]

---

[54] This is shaped like an inverted cup with feet and a head lying in the left rib-side.

[55] This may be as large as an arm lying from above the umbilicus possibly up to the heart.

[56] This is shaped like an inverted plate lying in the upper abdomen.

Accumulation of the lungs is called rushing breath.[57] Accumulation of the kidneys is called running piglet.[58] People call it qi lump. Dan-xi explained that a lump has a physical form, while qi is not able to produce (such) form. Both are phlegm or food accumulation or dead blood. If they lie in the center, they are phlegm accumulation. If they are located on the right side, they are food accumulation. If they are on the left side, they are dead blood. Lumps in women's abdomens are, in most cases, dead blood. Those which are immovable are called concretion. Those which are movable are called conglomeration.

Their great (treatment) methods are to soften with salty (medicinals) and to whittle down with hard (medicinals), and the ruling (formulas) are those which move the qi and open phlegm. One may use *Kui Jian Tang* (Open Hardness Decoction) and *Kui Jian Wan* (Open Hardness Pills) to treat them. Externally, apply *Hu Po Gao* (Amber Paste) and *San Sheng Gao* (Three Sages Paste).

*Kui Jian Tang* (Open Hardness Decoction)

*Kui Jian Tang* is composed of *Zhi Shi* (Fructus Immaturus Citri Aurantii), *Dang Gui* (Radix Angelicae Sinensis), *Ban Xia* (Rhizoma Pinelliae Ternatae), *Chen Pi* (Pericarpium Citri Reticulatae), *Bai Zhu* (Rhizoma Atractylodis Macrocephalae), *Xiang Fu* (Rhizoma Cyperi Rotundi), *Hou Po* (Cortex Magnoliae Officinalis), *Shan Zha* (Fructus Crataegi), *Sha Ren* (Fructus Amomi), and *Mu Xiang* (Radix Auklandiae Lappae). If there is a lump in the left rib-side, add *Qing Pi* (Pericarpium Citri Reticulatae Viride). If there is a lump in the right rib-side, add *E Zhu* (Rhizoma Curcumae Zedoariae). In case of blood lumps, add *Tao Ren* (Semen Pruni Persicae), *Hong Hua* (Flos Carthami Tinctorii), and *Rou Gui* (Cortex Cinnamomi Cassiae) and remove *Ban Xia* (Rhizoma Pinelliae Ternatae). In case of food accumulation lumps, add *Shen Qu* (Massa Medica Fermentata). In case of phlegm lumps, add *Hai Fu Shi* (Pumice) and *Gua*

---

[57] This is shaped like an inverted cup lying in the right rib-side.

[58] This starts from the lower abdomen, rushing upward, possibly surging into the heart or the throat.

*Lou* (Fructus Trichosanthis Kirlowii) and remove *Shan Zha* (Fructus Crataegi). For thin persons, add a small amount of *Ren Shen* (Radix Panacis Ginseng).

*Kui Jian Wan* (Open Hardness Pills)

This is *Kui Jian Tang* plus *Hai Shi* (Pumice), *Wa Leng Zi* (Concha Arcae), and *Bie Jia* (Carapax Amydae Sinensis). Powder (these medicinals) together and mix with *A Wei* (Resina Ferulae Asafoetidae) melted by boiling in vinegar. Then make this into pills the size of firmiana seeds with rice cooked in ginger juice. Administer 60 pills each time with yellow (*i.e.*, rice) wine.

*Hu Po Gao* (Amber Paste)

Powder equal amounts of *Da Huang* (Radix Et Rhizoma Rhei) and *Mang Xiao* (Mirabilitum) and pound them with leeks into a paste. Apply this, fixing it (in place) with a thread. Once the nose smells its odor, it will bring effect.

*San Sheng Gao* (Three Sages Paste)

Powder one half catty of *Sheng Shi Hui* (Calx Viva) and stir-fry it in a pottery container till it becomes light red in color. Then remove from the fire. When it becomes a little cool, put in one *liang* of powdered *Da Huang* (Radix Et Rhizoma Rhei) and stir-fry together without the fire. When (the container) becomes still cooler, put in five *qian* of powdered *Gui Xin* (Cortex Rasus Cinnamomi). Stir-fry this for awhile, and then put in vinegar. Stir these (over the fire) till they become a black paste. Spread a thick smear of this paste (over the affected area) after heating.

## 30. The Five Taxations & Six Extremes Are All Due to Fire Scorching the Heavenly True

The five taxations mean taxation damage of the five viscera. The six extremes refer to parched skin, shedding of the flesh, sinew wilting, heaviness of the bones, desiccated fluids, and a rapid pulse. These pathoconditions are mostly seen in taxed and timid persons. They are all due to the two fires[59] which run out of control. Because (these fires) boil and scorch the heavenly true, the qi and blood, essence and spirit are debilitated and weakened day by day. Therefore, the six extremes arise.

(To decide on) a method for treating taxation, one should detect which of the viscera is vacuous and which is replete, identifying qi vacuity, blood vacuity, qi heat, and blood heat. Only with true knowledge and penetrating insight can one treat without a mistake. When a viscus is vacuous, its pulse must be vacuous and small. If a viscus is replete, its pulse must be replete and large. Qi vacuity exhibits a white face with no spirit. Blood vacuity exhibits a black and desiccated, thin face. Those suffering from qi heat have a red, glossy face, and a loud and clear voice. Their disease worsens during the day, and their pulse is floating and rapid. Those suffering from blood heat have a red but dark face and a loud but turbid voice. Their disease worsens during the night, and their pulse is deep and rapid. If there is heat in both the qi and blood, the disease remains serious (all the time,) during the day and the night. There is rapid breathing with desiccated fluids. Going by these (criteria,) one will never fail to hit (the mark).

For qi vacuity, use *Si Jun Tang* (Four Gentlemen Decoction). For blood vacuity, use *Si Wu Tang* (Four Materials Decoction). For vacuity of both the qi and blood, use *Ba Zhen Tang* (Eight Pearls Decoction). To clear qi, use *Mai Dong* (Tuber Ophiopogonis Japonici), *Zhu Ye* (Folium Bambusae), *Yin Hua* (Flos Lonicerae Japonicae), *Chai Hu* (Radix Bupleuri), *Zhi Mu* (Rhizoma Anemarrhenae Asphodeloidis), and the like. To cool the blood, use *Tian Dong* (Tuber Asparagi Cochinensis), *Sheng Di* (uncooked Radix Rehmanniae), *Hu Huang Lian* (Rhizoma Picrorrhizae), *Huang Bai* (Cortex

---

[59] *I. e.*, ministerial fire and sovereign fire.

Phellodendri), *Huang Qin* (Radix Scutellariae Baicalensis), and the like. To quiet the heart spirit, use *Fu Shen* (Sclerotium Pararadicis Poriae Cocos), *Yuan Zhi* (Radix Polygalae Tenuifoliae), *Suan Zao Ren* (Semen Zizyphi Spinosae), and the like. To strengthen the sinews and bones, use *Niu Xi* (Radix Achyranthis Bidentatae), *Du Zhong* (Cortex Eucommiae Ulmoidis), *Hu Gu* (Os Tigridis), and the like. To supplement yang, use *Lu Rong* (Cornu Parvum Cervi), *Gou Qi Zi* (Fructus Lycii Chinensis), *Suo Yang* (Herba Cynomorii Songarici), *Rou Cong Rong* (Herba Cistanchis Deserticolae), *Tu Si Zi* (Semen Cuscutae Chinensis), and the like. To supplement yin, use *Shan Yao* (Radix Dioscoreae Oppositae), *Dan Pi* (Cortex Radicis Moutan), *Gui Ban* (Plastrum Testudinis), *Bai Zi Ren* (Semen Biotae Orientalis), and the like. To downbear ministerial fire, use *Huang Bai* (Cortex Phellodendri) and *Zhi Mu* (Rhizoma Anemarrhenae Asphodeloidis). To astringe essence, use *Long Gu* (Os Draconis), *Mu Li Fen* (powdered Concha Ostreae), *Lu Jiao Shuang* (Cornu Degelatinum Cervi), *Shan Zhu Yu* (Fructus Corni Officinalis), *Chu Shi Zi* (Fructus Broussonetiae), *Chi Shi Zhi* (Hallyositum Rubrum), and the like.

*Si Jun Tang* (Four Gentlemen Decoction) [See chapter 9.]

*Si Wu Tang* (Four Materials Decoction) [See chapter 10.]

*Ba Zhen Tang* (Eight Pearls Decoction) [See chapter 10.]

# 31. Blood Ejection Comes from the Bowel of the Stomach

Blood ejection (*i.e.,* hematemesis) comes from the stomach. The cause may be damage done by excessive drinking, damage done by carrying weights, damage from knocks and falls, damage done by taxation, excessive taxation of the heart, or qi counterflow provoked by violent anger. Since there are various causes, one must make a study of the pulse and a careful inquiry before meting out treatment.

The ruling (formula) is *Xi Jiao Di Huang Tang* (Rhinoceros Horn & Rehmannia Decoction). For wine damage, add *Ge Gen* (Radix Puerariae), *Huang Lian* (Rhizoma Coptidis Chinensis), *Mao Gen* (Rhizoma Imperatae Cylindricae), and *Ou Zhi* (Succus Rhizomatis Nelumbinis Nuciferae). For internal damage (caused by falls and knocks), add *Dang Gui* (Radix Angelicae Sinensis), *Tao Ren* (Semen Pruni Persicae), *Hong Hua* (Flos Carthami Tinctorii), and *Jiu Zhi* (Succus Allii Tuberosi). For sexual taxation, add *Dang Gui* (Radix Angelicae Sinensis), *Shu Di* (cooked Radix Rehmanniae), *Zhi Mu* (Rhizoma Anemarrhenae Asphodeloidis), *Huang Bai* (Cortex Phellodendri), *Zhi Zi* (Fructus Gardeniae Jasminoidis), and *Zhu Li* (Succus Bambusae). For taxation damage of the heart, add *Suan Zao Ren* (Semen Zizyphi Spinosae), *Fu Shen* (Sclerotium Pararadicis Poriae Cocos), *Xuan Shen* (Radix Scrophulariae Ningpoensis), and *Dang Gui* (Radix Angelicae Sinensis). For damage due to anger, add *Qing Dai* (Pulvis Indigonis) and *Huang Qin* (Radix Scutellariae Baicalensis). If the essence spirit is sound and strong but the stool is dry and bound with incessant ejection of blood, add stir-fried black *Da Huang* (Radix Et Rhizoma Rhei), mashed *Tao Ren* (Semen Pruni Persicae), and child's urine. If there is ejection of blood in large amounts, the physical body and looks are deprived of color, and the pulse is faint bordering on expiry, drink *Du Shen Tang* (Solitary Ginseng Decoction). This is the method of treating blood desertion by boosting the qi. When qi becomes effulgent, blood is engendered.

*Xi Jiao Di Huang Tang* (Rhinoceros Horn & Rehmannia Decoction)

*Xi Jiao Di Huang Tang* includes *Dan Pi* (Cortex Radicis Moutan) and *Chi Shao* (Radix Rubrus Paeoniae Lactiflorae). It is able to cure all (species of) blood loss, but, to make it good, one should make additions and subtractions.

# 32. The Root of Nosebleeding Is in the Lung Channel

In nose bleeding, blood exits through the nose. The nose is the orifice of the lungs. For that reason, (nose bleeding) is said to be rooted in the lung channel. To treat it, use *Ku Qin* (old Radix Scutellariae Baicalensis), *Mao Gen* (Rhizoma Imperatae Cylindricae), *Bai Ye* (Cacumen Biotae Orientalis), and *Ou Jie* (Nodus Rhizomatis Nelumbinis Nuciferae). Or pound seven pieces each of *He Ye Di* (Basis Folii Nelumbinis) and *Ou Jie* (Nodus Rhizomatis Nelumbinis Nuciferae), decoct them in water, and then administer.

# 33. Blood in Phlegm Drool Is Ascribed to the Spleen

Since phlegm is generated by the spleen, phlegm containing blood comes from the spleen. This requires *Xi Jiao Di Huang Tang* (Rhinoceros Horn & Rehmannia Decoction) plus *Bai Shao* (Radix Albus Paeoniae Lactiflorae), *Fu Ling* (Sclerotium Poriae Cocos), *Gua Lou Ren* (Semen Trichosanthis Kirlowii), and *Zhu Li* (Succus Bambusae). If the blood is blackish purple, add mashed *Tao Ren* (Semen Pruni Persicae), *Jiu Zhi* (Succus Allii Tuberosi), and *Dang Gui* (Radix Angelicae Sinensis).

# 34. Hacking & Spitting of Blood Are Ascribed to the Kidney Channel

Hacking of blood refers to hacking up specks of blood (*i.e.,* hemoptysis). Spitting of blood is fresh blood coming up with spitting (*i.e.,* hematemesis). Both are ascribed to the kidney channel. To treat these, add *Zhi Mu* (Rhizoma Anemarrhenae Asphodeloidis), *Huang Bai* (Cortex Phellodendri), *Xuan Shen* (Radix Scrophulariae Ningpoensis), and *Shu Di* (cooked Radix Rehmanniae) to *Xi Jiao Di Huang Tang* (Rhinoceros Horn & Rehmannia Decoction).

# 35. Gaping Gums Are Produced by Extreme Heat of the *Yang Ming*

Bleeding from the seams of the gums is called gaping gums. This is due to heat in the foot *yang ming* channel. The vessel of the *yang ming* travels through the upper gums. The vessel of the hand *yang ming* travels through the lower gums. When damp heat of the *yang ming* steams upward, the gums putrefy and bleed. (To treat this,) decoct and administer *Huang Qin* (Radix Scutellariae Baicalensis), *Lian Qiao* (Fructus Forsythiae Suspensae), *Bo He* (Herba Menthae Haplocalysis), *Zhi Zi* (Fructus Gardeniae Jasminoidis), and *Gan Cao* (Radix Glycyrrhizae).

Externally, stir-fry *Bai Cao Shuang* (Pulvis Fumi Carbonisati) and *Long Gu* (Os Draconis) with salt, powder, and then apply.

# 36. Tongue Bleeding Arises from the Fire of the *Shao Yin*

Bleeding from the surface of the tongue is called tongue bleeding. (To treat it,), dab powdered stir-fried *Huai Hua* (Flos Sophorae Japonicae) (on the affected area). If the tongue is so enlarged as to protrude out of the mouth, applying *Bing Pian* (Borneol) is instantly effective.

# 37. Abdominal Constriction Is Classified into Phlegm & Fire

If a fat person feels constriction inside their abdomen, this is due to damp phlegm streaming into the stomach. It requires *Cang Zhu* (Rhizoma Atractylodis) and *Xiang Fu* (Rhizoma Cyperi Rotundi) to dry rheum and move the qi. If a thin person feels constriction inside their abdomen, this is due to heat qi fuming and steaming the stomach. It requires *Cang Zhu* (Rhizoma Atractylodis) and *Huang Lian* (Rhizoma Coptidis Chinensis) to open depression and clear heat.

# 38. Vexatious Heat in the Chest Can be Divided into Vacuity & Repletion

(In regard to) vexatious heat in the chest, if it is repletion heat, it is necessary to use *Zhi Zi Ren* (Fructus Gardeniae Jasminoidis). If it is vacuity vexation, it is necessary to use *Ren Shen* (Radix Panacis Ginseng), *Bai Zhu* (Rhizoma Atractylodis Macrocephalae), *Fu Ling* (Sclerotium Poriae Cocos), *Huang Qin* (Radix Scutellariae Baicalensis), *Bai Shao* (Radix Albus Paeoniae Lactiflorae), and *Mai Dong* (Tuber Ophiopogonis Japonici).

# 39. Fright Palpitations Are
# the Result of Confounding Phlegm & Fear

Fright palpitations are due to phlegm confounding the orifices of the heart which is, (in turn,) usually caused by fear. To treat this, use *Er Chen Tang* (Two Aged [Ingredients] Decoction) plus *Fu Shen* (Sclerotium Pararadicis Poriae Cocos), *Yuan Zhi* (Radix Polygalae Tenuifoliae), *Dang Gui* (Radix Angelicae Sinensis), *Bai Zi Ren* (Semen Biotae Orientalis), *Suan Zao Ren* (Semen Zizyphi Spinosae), and *Ren Shen* (Radix Panacis Ginseng). Or use *Ba Wu Ding Zhi Wan* (Eight Materials Stabilize Mind Pills) or *Bu Xin Dan* (Supplement the Heart Elixir).

*Er Chen Tang* (Two Aged [Ingredients] Decoction) [See chapter 11.]

*Ba Wu Ding Zhi Wan* (Eight Materials Stabilize the Mind Pills)

*Ba Wu Ding Zhi* quiets the heart and spirit, settles fright, and supplements the qi. It is composed of *Niu Huang* (Calculus Bovis), *Ren Shen* (Radix Panacis Ginseng), *Yuan Zhi* (Radix Polygalae Tenuifoliae), *Fu Shen* (Sclerotium Pararadicis Poriae Cocos), *Chang Pu* (Rhizoma Acori Graminei), *Fu Ling* (Sclerotium Poriae Cocos), *Bai Zhu* (Rhizoma Atractylodis Macrocephalae), and *Mai Dong* (Tuber Ophiopogonis Japonici). Make these into pills with honey, coat with *Zhu Sha* (Cinnabar), and administer.

*Bu Xin Dan* (Supplement the Heart Elixir)

*Bu Xin Dan* is a legacy left by our predecessors. It is able to treat fright palpitations and difficulty sleeping. It is composed of *Dang Gui* (Radix Angelicae Sinensis), *Sheng Di* (uncooked Radix Rehmanniae), *Tian Dong* (Tuber Asparagi Cochinensis), *Mai Dong* (Tuber Ophiopogonis Japonici), *Suan Zao Ren* (Semen Zizyphi Spinosae), *Bai Zi Ren* (Semen Biotae Orientalis), *Yuan Zhi* (Radix Polygalae Tenuifoliae), *Dan Shen* (Radix Salviae Miltiorrhizae), *Ren Shen* (Radix Panacis Ginseng), *Yuan Shen* (Radix Scrophulariae Ningpoensis), *Fu Ling* (Sclerotium Poriae Cocos), *Jie Geng* (Radix Platycodi Grandiflori), and *Wu Wei Zi* (Fructus Schisandrae Chinensis) made into pills.

# 40. Impaired Memory Is a Product of Shortage of Blood Due to Anxiety & Depression

The disease of impaired memory (*i.e.*, forgetfulness) is due to excessive anxiety and thought damaging the pericardium. Since the abode of the spirit is not clear, the person is liable to forget in a blink. The appropriate (formulas) are *Gui Pi Tang* (Return the Spleen Decoction) and *Ba Wu Ding Zhi Wan* (Eight Materials Stabilize Mind Pills).

*Gui Pi Tang* (Return the Spleen Decoction)

*Gui Pi Tang* includes *Si Jun* (Four Gentlemen [Decoction]) plus *Mu Xiang* (Radix Auklandiae Lappae), stir-fried *Huang Qi* (Radix Astragali Membranacei), *Yuan Zhi* (Radix Polygalae Tenuifoliae), *Zao Ren* (Semen Zizyphi Spinosae), *Yuan Rou* (Arillus Euphoriae Longanae), *Dang Gui* (Radix Angelicae Sinensis), *Jiang* (Rhizoma Zingiberis), and *Da Zao* (Fructus Zizyphi Jujubae). It is divinely (*i.e.*, miraculously) effective for impaired memory.

# 41. Mania & Withdrawal Are Divided into Extreme Heat of the Heart & Liver

When there is extreme heat in the heart, withdrawal arises. If there is extreme heat in the liver, mania arises. Withdrawal is usually characterized by joy (*i.e.*, excitation) and mania by anger. If the pulse is floating and large, this is favorable. If it is deep and thin, this is unfavorable. Withdrawal requires clearing the heart and nurturing the spirit with *Ning Zhi Hua Tan Tang* (Calm Mind & Transform Phlegm Decoction) as the ruling (formula). Mania requires dispelling wind and eliminating heat with *Fang Feng Tong Sheng San* (Notopterygium Sage-communicated Powder) as the ruling (formula).

*Ning Zhi Hua Tan Tang* (Calm the Mind & Transform Phlegm Decoction)

*Ning Zhi Hua Tan* is composed of *Ren Shen* (Radix Panacis Ginseng), *Tian Ma* (Rhizoma Gastrodiae Elatae), *Huang Lian* (Rhizoma Coptidis Chinensis), *Dan Xing* (bile-processed Rhizoma Arisaematis), *Fu Ling* (Sclerotium Poriae Cocos), *Chen Pi* (Pericarpium Citri Reticulatae), *Ban Xia* (Rhizoma Pinelliae Ternatae), *Zao Ren* (Semen Zizyphi Spinosae), and *Chang Pu Gen* (Rhizoma Acori Graminei).

*Kai Mi San* (Open Confounding Powder)

If a woman suffers from withdrawal or mania, (use) *Tao Ren* (Semen Pruni Persicae), *Chi Shao* (Radix Rubrus Paeoniae Lactiflorae), *Dang Gui* (Radix Angelicae Sinensis), *Chai Hu* (Radix Bupleuri), *Fu Ling* (Sclerotium Poriae Cocos), *Gan Cao* (Radix Glycyrrhizae), *Yuan Zhi* (Radix Polygalae Tenuifoliae), *Bai Zhu* (Rhizoma Atractylodis Macrocephalae), *Su Mu* (Lignum Sappan), and *Sheng Di* (uncooked Radix Rehmanniae).

*Fang Feng Tong Sheng San* (Notopterygium Sage-communicated Powder) [See #7 above.]

# 42. In Epilepsy, One Should Detect Serious & Slight Phlegm & Fire

Generally speaking, epilepsy is ascribed to phlegm, fire, and fright, and there is no need to divide it into five categories[60] in terms of its treatment. In general, the ruling (method) is to move phlegm with *Huang Lian* (Rhizoma Coptidis Chinensis), *Nan Xing* (Rhizoma Arisaematis), *Gua Lou* (Fructus Trichosanthis Kirlowii), and *Ban Xia* (Rhizoma Pinelliae Ternatae). To treat it, one should find out (which is the cause,) phlegm or fire, and determine its amounts. Then one can accomplish cures without fail. If there is heat, use cool medicinals to clear the heart. If there is phlegm, it is necessary to use ejecting medicinals (*i.e.*, emetics). After

---

[60] The five traditional categories of epilepsy are goat, horse, cow, swine, and chicken epilepsy. In another classification, dog epilepsy is substituted for horse epilepsy. These categories are determined by the noise the patient makes during the attack.

ejection, use *An Shen Wan* (Quiet the Spirit Pills) and medicinals for leveling the liver, such as *Chai Hu* (Radix Bupleuri), *Qing Dai* (Pulvis Indigonis), and *Chuan Xiong* (Radix Ligustici Wallichii).

*An Shen Wan* (Quiet the Spirit Pills)

*An Shen Wan* are composed of *Zhu Sha* (Cinnabar), *Gan Cao* (Radix Glycyrrhizae), *Dang Gui* (Radix Angelicae Sinensis), *Huang Lian* (Rhizoma Coptidis Chinensis), and *Sheng Di Huang* (uncooked Radix Rehmanniae). Their effect on epilepsy is quite commendable.

# 43. Turbid Urine Is Divided into Red & White

Turbid urine is due to heat of the small intestine channel bound in the urinary bladder. If there is blood heat, (the urine) is reddish. If there is qi heat, it is white. To treat this, use *Qing Xin Lian Zi Yin* (Clear the Heart Lotus Seed Drink). In case of reddish (urine), add *Mu Tong* (Caulis Akebiae) and *Huang Bai* (Cortex Phellodendri). In case of white (urine), add *Chi Ling* (Sclerotium Rubrus Cocos) and *Hua Shi* (Talcum).

*Qing Xin Lian Zi Yin* (Clear the Heart Lotus Seed Drink)

*Qing Xin* includes *Lian Zi* (Semen Nelumbinis Nuciferae), *Huang Qin* (Radix Scutellariae Baicalensis), *Che Qian Zi* (Semen Plantaginis), *Chai Hu* (Radix Bupleuri), *Di Gu Pi* (Cortex Radicis Lycii Chinensis), *Ren Shen* (Radix Panacis Ginseng), *Mai Dong* (Tuber Ophiopogonis Japonici), *Chi Fu Ling* (Sclerotium Rubrus Poriae Cocos), *Huang Qi* (Radix Astragali Membranacei), and *Gan Cao* (Radix Glycyrrhizae). Taking it makes turbid urine clear.

*Bei Xie Fen Qing Yin* (Dioscorea Hypoglauca Separate the Clear Drink)

In *Bei Xie Fen Qing Yin*, there are *Wu Yao* (Radix Linderae Strychnifoliae) and *Chang Pu* (Rhizoma Acori Graminei), *Gan Cao Shao* (Tenuis Radicis Glycyrrhizae), and *Yi Zhi* (Fructus Alpiniae Oxyphyllae) standing side by side with *Fu Ling* (Sclerotium Poriae Cocos).

# 44. Sweating May Be Called
# (Either) Spontaneous or Night

Spontaneous sweating is constant, moderate sweating for no reason. It becomes massive on movement. This is ascribed to yang vacuity. Night sweats are sweating during sleep which stops on waking. This is ascribed to yin vacuity. Spontaneous sweating requires supplementing yang and regulating the defensive. Night sweats requires supplementing yin and downbearing fire. For spontaneous sweating, use *Bu Zhong Yi Qi Tang* (Supplement the Center & Boost the Qi Decoction) plus *Ma Huang Gen* (Radix Ephedrae) and *Fu Xiao Mai* (Semen Levis Tritici Aestivi). In case of severe vacuity, add one or two pieces of *Shu Fu Zi* (Radix Lateralis Praeparatus Aconiti Carmichaeli). Within this formula, *Sheng Ma* (Rhizoma Cimicifugae) and *Chai Hu* (Radix Bupleuri) should be stir-fried with honey to suppress their lifting and effusing nature. They must be used, however, for no others but they can lead *Ren Shen* (Radix Panacis Ginseng) and *Huang Qi* (Radix Astragali Membranacei) to the muscular (*i.e.*, fleshy) exterior. For night sweats, use *Dang Gui Liu Huang Tang* (Rehmannia Six Yellows Decoction).

*Dang Gui Liu Huang Tang* (Rehmannia Six Yellows Decoction)

*Liu Huang Tang* is a good formula for night sweats. It is composed of seven flavors: *Dang Gui* (Radix Angelicae Sinensis), *Sheng Di* (uncooked Radix Rehmanniae), *Shu Di* (cooked Radix Rehmanniae), *Huang Bai* (Cortex Phellodendri), *Huang Lian* (Rhizoma Coptidis Chinensis), wine stir-fried *Huang Qin* (Radix Scutellariae Baicalensis), and *Huang Qi* (Radix Astragali Membranacei).

*Du Sheng San* (Single Sage Powder)

*Du Sheng San* (Single Sage Powder) is composed of *Wu Bei Zi* (Galla Rhois Chinensis). Powder, mix with saliva, and apply it to the umbilicus for one night. Once sweat exits, relief ensues.

*Bu Zhong Yi Qi Tang* (Supplement the Center & Boost the Qi Decoction) [See #5 above.]

# 45. The Nine Kinds of Heart Pain Are Located in the Stomach Duct

Heart pain is pain in the stomach duct. In olden times, heart pain was divided into nine categories. The first is worms. The second is infixation.[61] The third is wind. The fourth is palpitations. The fifth is rheum. The sixth is food. The seventh is cold. The eighth is heat. The ninth is coming and going (*i.e.*, intermittent) pain. I have made a study of this classification. However, although there are (these various) names, no one has given any explanations of them. Therefore, physicians have difficulty in identifying and treating them. Since I have gained (some) knowledge (of this), I cannot refrain from demonstrating it to later students.

Worm pain is anguish and disquietude with vomiting of clear water and a crab-legs pattern on the face. (To treat this,) use *Bai Fan* (Alum), *Xiong Huang* (Realgar), and *Bing Lang* (Semen Arecae Catechu). Powder these and administer with boiled water. Infixation pain is heart pain which is absent at ordinary times but arises suddenly with raving and delirious speech and a pulse which comes sometimes large and sometimes small. (To treat this,) decoct in water and take one *liang* of *Yin Hua* (Flos Lonicerae Japonicae). Wind pain is caused by wind evils entering the spleen while sleeping in the open during summer days. It is a spleen pain linking to the heart. It goes up and down irregularly, usually accompanied by retching and vomiting. (To treat it), use *Huo Xiang Zheng Qi San* (Agastache Correct the Qi Powder). Palpitation pain is a slight pain, a feeling of dull pain in the chest. This is due to fright wind overwhelming the heart. To treat it, use *Er Chen Tang* (Two Aged [Ingredients] Decoction) plus *Fu Shen* (Sclerotium Pararadicis Poriae Cocos), *Yuan Zhi* (Radix Polygalae Tenuifoliae), *Huang Lian* (Rhizoma Coptidis Chinensis), *Zhi Shi* (Fructus Immaturus Citri Aurantii), and *Dang Gui* (Radix Angelicae Sinensis). Rheum pain is caused by phlegm rheum lodging in the stomach duct. Because there is obstruction, qi counterflows. As a result, pain arises. The (sick) person invariably has a sooty color below their eyes and suffers

---

[61] This refers to malign stroke. It is a syndrome of alternating fever and chills and derangement.

from icy water collecting in the chest. For a serious case, use *Gun Tan Wan* (Roll Phlegm Pills) to precipitate. For a slight case, use *Dao Tan Tang* (Abduct Phlegm Decoc-tion) plus *Cang Zhu* (Rhizoma Atractylodis), *Xiang Fu* (Rhizoma Cyperi Rotundi), and *Chuan Xiong* (Radix Ligustici Wallichii). Food pain is glomus and fullness in the chest, possibly accompanied by eructation, acid regurgitation, and aversion to the smell of food. (To treat it,) use *Ping Wei San* (Calm the Stomach Powder) adding *Zhi Shi* (Fructus Immaturus Citri Aurantii), *Shan Zha* (Fructus Crataegi), *Lai Fu Zi* (Semen Raphani Sativi), *Shen Qu* (Massa Medica Fermentata), *Mai Ya* (Fructus Germinatus Hordei Vulgaris), and the like. Cold pain is due to visiting cold assaulting the stomach. The pain may be violent with cold limbs and the pulse is deep and slow. The ruling (formula for it) is *Pan Cong San* (Scallion Powder).

Heat pain is due to heat accumulation in the stomach. It is accompanied by heart vexation, generalized fever, and inhibited defecation and urination. (To treat it,) use *Er Chen Tang* (Two Aged [Ingredients] Decoction) plus *Zhi Zi* (Fructus Gardeniae Jasminoidis), *Huang Lian* (Rhizoma Coptidis Chinensis), *Chuan Xiong* (Radix Ligustici Wallichii), and *Xiang Fu* (Rhizoma Cyperi Rotundi).

Coming and going pain is intermittent pain with a red facial complexion and thirst. Thin persons are liable to this disease. It is pain caused by stomach fire. (To treat it,) add *Zhi Zi* (Fructus Gardeniae Jasminoidis), *Xiang Fu* (Rhizoma Cyperi Rotundi), and *Chen Pi* (Pericarpium Citri Reticulatae) to *Si Wu Tang* (Four Materials Decoction).

Dan-xi said:

> If a person likes eating hot food, the stomach opening will be damaged. Then clear blood exits and is held up so as to produce blood stasis. (This blood stasis) gathers and accumulates in the stomach, often giving rise to heart pain. Its symptoms include exacerbation of the pain on having hot beverage. The pulse is deep and choppy.

For a serious case, prescribe *Tao Ren Cheng Qi Tang* (Persica Order the Qi Decoction) to precipitate (blood stasis). For a slight case, use *Si Wu Tang* (Four Materials Decoction) plus *Tao Ren* (Semen Pruni Persicae), *Hong Hua*

(Flos Carthami Tinctorii), *Ru Xiang* (Resina Olibani), *Mo Yao* (Resina Myrrhae), *Wu Ling Zhi* (Feces Trogopterori Seu Pteromi), *Yuan Hu* (Rhizoma Corydalis Yanhusuo), and the like.

*Pan Cong San* (Scallion Powder)

*Pan Cong San* (Scallion Powder) is composed of *Fu Ling* (Sclerotium Poriae Cocos), *Bing Lang* (Semen Arecae Catechu), *Pao Jiang* (blast-fried Rhizoma Zingiberis), *Sha Ren* (Fructus Amomi), mix-fried *Gan Cao* (Radix Glycyrrhizae), *Rou Gui* (Cortex Cinnamomi Cassiae), *San Leng* (Rhizoma Spargani), *Qing Pi* (Pericarpium Citri Reticulatae Viride), *Ding Pi* (Cortex Caryophylli), *Cang Zhu* (Rhizoma Atractylodis), *Yuan Hu* (Rhizoma Corydalis Yanhusuo), and *E Zhu* (Rhizoma Curcumae Zedoariae). It treats heart pain and mounting (*i.e.*, *shan*) pain. (This is taken with scallion.)

*Huo Xiang Zheng Qi San* (Agastache Correct the Qi Powder) [See #19, above.]

*Gun Tan Wan* (Roll Phlegm Pills) [See #12 above.]

*Er Chen Tang* (Two Aged [Ingredients] Decoction) [See chapter 11.]

*Dao Tan Tang* (Abduct Phlegm Decoction) [See chapter 11.]

*Si Wu Tang* (Four Materials Decoction) [See chapter 10.]

*Ping Wei San* (Calm the Stomach Powder) [See chapter 13.]
*Tao Ren Cheng Qi Tang* (Persica Order the Qi Decoction) [See #3 above.]

# 46. The Seven Categories of Mounting Qi Are Diseases of the *Jue Yin*

The seven categories of mounting (*i.e.*, *shan*) are cold, water, blood, qi, sinew, foxy, and bulging mounting. Zhang Zi-he has given these a detailed explanation. Dan-xi said, "Mounting is exclusively ruled by the liver channel, having nothing to do with the kidney channel." Its cause is usually damp heat qi of the liver channel pouring downward. Because it is unable to drain or skip out, it causes unilateral sagging (of the testicles) or mounting pain.

Once I designed a formula to treat this. Not more than three or four doses of it can bring magical results. It has hit 100 out of 100 occurrences, responding well without a fail. (I) call it *San Jie Tang* (Three Rapids Decoction).

*San Jie Tang* (Three Rapids Decoction)

(This formula is composed of) *Qing Pi* (Pericarpium Citri Reticulatae Viride), one *qian*; *Guan Gui* (tubiform Cortex Cinnamomi Cassiae), five *fen*; *Gui Wei* (Extremitas Radicis Angelicae Sinensis), one *qian*; *Bing Lang* (Semen Arecae Catechu), two *qian*; *Da Hui Xiang* (Fructus Anisi Stellati), seven *fen*, stir-fried a little; *Huang Bai* (Cortex Phellodendri), three *fen*; *Ju He* (Semen Citri), two *qian*; *Mu Tong* (Caulis Akebiae), two *qian*; *Zi Su* (Fructus Perillae Frutescentis), seven *fen*; *Xiang Fu* (Rhizoma Cyperi Rotundi), one *qian*; *Chi Fu Ling* (Sclerotium Rubrus Poriae Cocos), two *qian*; *Chai Hu* (Radix Bupleuri), one *qian*; *Li Zhi He* (Semen Litchi Sinensis), seven pieces, stir-fried; and *Jiang* (Rhizoma Zingiberis), one slice. Boil these in three bowls of water down to one bowlful. Administer hot on an empty stomach.

# 47. Rib-side Pain Differs on the Two Sides[62]

Rib-side pain is pain in the region of the rib-side. The rib-sides are ascribed to the *shao yang* gallbladder channel. If, in this region, phlegm rheum streams or static blood collects and accumulates, the qi will be unable to circulate and, hence, pain arises. With phlegm, the pulse is bowstring and slippery. With blood (stasis), the pulse is bowstring and

---

[62] It may seem that the discussion below does not discuss the difference between the left and the right rib-side pain, but instead the author talks of different treatments for food, blood, etc. problems. However, one should note that dead blood accumulates on the left side, while food accumulation lies on the right.

choppy. In case of phlegm, use *Chen Pi* (Pericarpium Citri Reticulatae), *Fu Ling* (Sclerotium Poriae Cocos), *Gua Lou* (Fructus Trichosanthis Kirlowii), *Gan Cao* (Radix Glycyrrhizae), *Zhi Ke* (Fructus Citri Aurantii), *Chai Hu* (Radix Bupleuri), *Bai Jie Zi* (Semen Sinapis Albae), *Zhu Li* (Succus Bambusae), and *Jiang Zhi* (Succus Rhizomatis Zingiberis). In case of blood (stasis), use *Dang Gui* (Radix Angelicae Sinensis), *Chi Shao* (Radix Rubrus Paeoniae Lactiflorae), *Tao Ren* (Semen Pruni Persicae), *Hong Hua* (Flos Carthami Tinctorii), *Chai Hu* (Radix Bupleuri), *Guan Gui* (tubiform Cortex Cinnamomi Cassiae), *Xiang Fu* (Rhizoma Cyperi Rotundi), and *Mo Yao* (Resina Myrrhae). If pain is caused by liver fire, add *Huang Lian* (Rhizoma Coptidis Chinensis) and *Long Dan Cao* (Radix Gentianae Scabrae). If pain is caused by food accumulation, add *Mai Ya* (Fructus Germinatus Hordei Vulgaris) and *Sha Ren* (Fructus Amomi).

# 48. Head Wind Is Divided into Left & Right

The head is the top of the body, subject to wind cold. When there is a chance, wind evils will intrude. If blood is vacuous and wind evils assault, then pain will arise on the left side (of the head). If the qi is vacuous and wind evils assault, pain will arise on the right side. If the pulse is floating and slippery, it is easy to treat. If the pulse is short and choppy, it is difficult to treat. The ruling formula is *Chuan Xiong Cha Tiao San* (Ligusticum & Tea Mixed Powder). In case of blood vacuity, add *Shu Di* (cooked Radix Rehmanniae) and *Dang Gui* (Radix Angelicae Sinensis). In case of qi vacuity, add *Huang Qi* (Radix Astragali Membranacei) and *Ren Shen* (Radix Panacis Ginseng). If there is phlegm, add *Ban Xia* (Rhizoma Pinelliae Ternatae) and *Nan Xing* (Rhizoma Arisaematis). If there is heat, add *Huang Qin* (Radix Scutellariae Baicalensis) and *Shi Gao* (Gypsum Fibrosum). In case of exuberant wind, add *Tian Ma* (Rhizoma Gastrodiae Elatae) and *Man Jing Zi* (Fructus Viticis). The method is (actually) to use the added medicinals as the ruling (ingredients), and the (standard) medicinals in this formula as the assistants.

*Chuan Xiong Cha Tiao San* (Ligusticum & Tea Mixed Powder)

*Chuan Xiong Cha Tiao San* is composed of eight flavors, (including) *Jing Jie* (Herba Schizonepetae Tenuifoliae), *Bo He* (Herba Menthae Haplocalysis), *Bai Zhi* (Radix Angelicae Dahuricae), *Fang Feng* (Radix Ledebouriellae Divaricatae), *Gan Cao* (Radix Glycyrrhizae), *Xi Xin* (Herba Asari Cum Radice), and *Qiang Huo* (Radix Et Rhizoma Notopterygii). It relieves head wind pain.

*Du Liang Wan* (Angelica Pills) [treats sudden contraction of wind cold with stiffness of and inability to turn round the head and the nape of the neck. This is popularly known as crick in the neck. It can treat any kind (of headache)].

*Xiang Bai Zhi* (Radix Angelicae Dahuricae), two *liang*. Grind into fine powder, mix with honey, and make into pills the size of a catapult pellet. Take one pill each time, chewing thoroughly before swallowing down with tea water or *Jing Jie* (Herba Schizonepetae Tenuifoliae) soup.

## 49. Lumbago Is Due to Kidney Vacuity or Wrenching & Contusion

The lumbus is the mansion of the kidneys where the major joints of the body are located. If there is excessive sexual taxation, then the kidneys become vacuous. If there is wrenching and contusion, then qi counter-flows. Detriment and damage due to carrying weights leads to congealed blood. Sleeping in a damp place subjects one to cold dampness. All these are causes of lumbago, and its manifestations differ depending upon the disease causes. Kidney vacuity gives a constant, mild pain, and the pulse is deep, bowstring, and large. Wrenching and contusion makes it difficult to bend (the lumbus) either forward or backward, and the pulse is deep, bowstring, and replete. Blood congelation gives a pain as if pricked by an awl, which is milder by day but worse by night. Damp heat is revealed by yellow urine and sloppy stools, and the pulse is deep, bowstring, fine, and rapid. Cold dampness is characterized by a pain arising in wet weather or after having sat for a long time.

In case of kidney vacuity, use *Dang Gui* (Radix Angelicae Sinensis), *Shu Di* (cooked Radix Rehmanniae), *Gou Qi* (Fructus Lycii Chinensis), *Niu Xi* (Radix Achyranthis Bidentatae), *Du Zhong* (Cortex Eucommiae Ulmoidis), *Hui Xiang* (Fructus Foeniculi Vulgaris), *Zhi Mu* (Rhizoma Anemarrhenae Asphodeloidis), *Huang Bai* (Cortex Phellodendri), *Xu Duan* (Radix Dipsaci), *Du Huo* (Radix Angelicae Pubescentis), and so on. In case of wrenching and contusion, use *Hui Xiang* (Fructus Foeniculi Vulgaris), *Mu Xiang* (Radix Auklandiae Lappae), *Chuan Xiong* (Radix Ligustici Wallichii), *Guan Gui* (tubiform Cortex Cinnamomi Cassiae), *Sha Ren* (Fructus Amomi), *Zhi Ke* (Fructus Citri Aurantii), and so on. In case of blood congelation, use *Gui Wei* (Extremitas Radicis Angelicae Sinensis), *Tao Ren* (Semen Pruni Persicae), *Hong Hua* (Flos Carthami Tinctorii), *Su Mu* (Lignum Sappan), *Ru Xiang* (Resina Olibani), *Mo Yao* (Resina Myrrhae), *Rou Gui* (Cortex Cinnamomi Cassiae), *Yuan Hu* (Rhizoma Corydalis Yanhusuo), *Du Huo* (Radix Angelicae Pubescentis), and so on. In case of damp heat, use *Fu Ling* (Sclerotium Poriae Cocos), *Bai Zhu* (Rhizoma Atractylodis Macrocephalae), *Chen Pi* (Pericarpium Citri Reticulatae), *Fang Ji* (Radix Stephaniae Tetrandrae), *Zhi Mu* (Rhizoma Anemarrhenae Asphodeloidis), *Fang Feng* (Radix Ledebouriellae Divaricatae), *Qin Jiao* (Radix Gentianae Macrophyllae), *Qiang Huo* (Radix Et Rhizoma Notopterygii), and so on. In case of cold dampness, use *Chuan Xiong* (Radix Ligustici Wallichii), *Dang Gui* (Radix Angelicae Sinensis), *Gui Zhi* (Ramulus Cinnamomi Cassiae), *Fu Zi* (Radix Lateralis Praeparatus Aconiti Carmichaeli), *Du Zhong* (Cortex Eucommiae Ulmoidis), *Niu Xi* (Radix Achyranthis Bidentatae), *Bai Zhi* (Radix Angelicae Dahuricae), *Cang Zhu* (Rhizoma Atractylodis), *Du Huo* (Radix Angelicae Pubescentis), and so on.

# 50. Abdominal Pain Is
# Due to Cold Qi or Food Stagnation

Central stomach duct pain is ascribed to the *tai yin*. Periumbilical abdominal pain is ascribed to the *shao yin*. Lower abdominal pain is ascribed to the *jue yin*. Constant, dull pain which gets neither better nor worse is due to cold. (Pain) arising and stopping irregularly is due to heat. Pain, which, once exacerbated, gives rise to desire to evacuate stools and which is relievable by evacuation, is due to food accumulation. Pain in a fixed place, immovable, is due to dead blood. Pain accompanied by inhibited urination and temporarily checkable by having acrid, pungent, and hot substances is due to phlegm. If, during attacks, pain makes lumps appear in the abdomen which immediately disappear when pressed with the hand and there is nausea and vomiting of clear water, this is due to worms. Pain arising on eating first hot and then cold food is due to lack of regulation between cold and heat. There is a true abdominal pain. When the pain attacks, there will appear a greenish blue sinew above the umbilicus. If the sinew penetrates up to the heart region, this is dangerous. If the philtrum is black, this is lethal. (In abdominal pain,) a thin, slow pulse is favorable, and a large, rapid pulse is unfavorable.

To treat (abdominal pain), use *Ping Wei San* (Calm the Stomach Powder) plus *Bai Shao* (Radix Albus Paeoniae Lactiflorae) as the ruling (formula). In case of cold, add *Gan Jiang* (dry Rhizoma Zingiberis), *Fu Zi* (Radix Lateralis Praeparatus Aconiti Carmichaeli), *Rou Gui* (Cortex Cinnamomi Cassiae), *Wu Zhu Yu* (Fructus Evodiae Rutecarpae), and the like. In case of heat, add *Bai Shao* (Radix Albus Paeoniae Lactiflorae) and *Huang Bai* (Cortex Phellodendri). If pain is severe, add *Chao Gan Jiang* (stir-fried dry Rhizoma Zingiberis). In case of food accumulation, add *Bing Lang* (Semen Arecae Catechu), *Zhi Shi* (Fructus Immaturus Citri Aurantii), *Shen Qu* Massa Medica Fermentata), *Mai Ya* (Fructus Germinatus Hordei Vulgaris), *Shan Zha* (Fructus Craetagi), *Lai Fu Zi* (Semen Raphani Sativi), and the like to disperse (food accumulation). If pain is severe, add *Da Huang* (Radix Et Rhizoma Rhei) and *Rou Gui* (Cortex Cinnamomi Cassiae) to precipitate. In case of dead blood, add *Gui Wei* (Extremitas Radicis Angelicae Sinensis), *Tao Ren* (Semen Pruni Persicae), *Wu Ling Zhi* (Feces Trogopterori Seu Pteromi), *Yuan Hu Suo* (Rhizoma Corydalis Yanhusuo), and the like to quicken (the blood). For a severe case, add *Da Huang* (Radix Et Rhizoma Rhei) and *Rou Gui* (Cortex Cinnamomi Cassiae) to precipitate. In case of damp phlegm, add *Nan Xing* (Rhizoma Arisaematis), *Ban Xia* (Rhizoma Pinelliae Ternatae), *Xiang Fu* (Rhizoma Cyperi Rotundi), *Fu Ling* (Sclerotium Poriae Cocos), *Zhi Ke* (Fructus Citri Aurantii), *Mu Tong* (Caulis Akebiae), and the like. For worm pain, add *Shi Jun Zi Rou* (Fructus Quisqualis Indicae) and *Ku Lian Gen Pi* (Cortex Radicis Meliae Azerdachis). In case of lack of regulation between cold and heat, add *Shao Yao* (Radix Paeoniae Lactiflorae), *Gui Zhi* (Ramulus Cinnamomi Cassiae), and *Da Huang* (Radix Et Rhizoma Rhei).

Abdominal pain linking to the rib-side with cold hands and feet and a hidden pulse is due to drink and food or phlegm rheum stopping up the extreme yin (*i.e., jue yin*), suppressing and obstructing the qi of the liver and gallbladder. The appropriate (treatment) is to seek ejection (by administering) boiled saltwater. This is a method of freeing depressed wood.

*Ping Wei San* (Calm the Stomach Powder) [See chapter 13.]

## 51. Wilting Is Due to Insufficiency & Damp Heat

The main idea of the *"Wei Lun* (Treatise on Wilting)*"* in the *Nei Jing (Inner Classic)* is as follows. Lung heat scorching the lobes results in weak, tense, thin skin and hair and crippling wilting arises. Heart qi heat gives rise to vessel wilting. (Therefore,) the sinews become slack and (one is) unable to stand on the earth. Liver qi heat gives rise to sinew wilting. (Thus) the ancestral sinew (*i.e.*, the penis) becomes slack. If spleen qi is hot, flesh wilting arises. Then the muscles and flesh become insensitive. Kidney qi heat results in bone wilting. (In that case,) the feet are unable to support the body.

The causes of wilting: It is very often (seen) that a long trip after disease, rising up (*i.e.*, going about) shortly after birthing, performance of bedroom affairs (*i.e.*, having sex) after extraordinarily felling (the body)[63], or (over)taxation damaging the bones and marrow result in both feet becoming wilted and limp. To treat (this) one should (use) medicinals to supplement the essence, nourish the blood, and strengthen the sinews and bones. In addition, (patients) must abstain from bedroom taxation if they intend to fully recover. The ruling (formula) is *Qi Wei Gu Zhen Wan* (Arouse Wilting & Secure the True Pills). If, during summer days when

---

[63] This implies grave intoxication.

damp heat is exuberant, one contracts damp heat evils and, hence, wilting, the appropriate (formula) is Li Dong-yuan's *Qing Zao Tang* (Clearing & Drying Decoction).

One person indulged in wine and, thus, was taken with wilting. I said (to him) that wine is a damp, hot substance. Since wine was responsible for wilting, (I) prescribed *Qing Zao Tang* (Clearing & Drying Decoction) with good effect.

*Qi Wei Gu Zhen Wan* (Arouse Wilting & Secure the True Pills)

(This formula is composed of) *Ren Shen* (Radix Panacis Ginseng), one *liang*; *Huang Qi* (Radix Astragali Membranacei), one *liang*; *Dang Gui* (Radix Angelicae Sinensis), two *liang*; *Niu Xi* (Radix Achyranthis Bidentatae), one and a half *liang*; *Rou Cong Rong* (Herba Cistanchis Deserticolae), stir-fried with wine, two *liang*; *Shu Di* (cooked Radix Rehmanniae), four *liang*; *Chuan Xiong* (Radix Ligustici Wallichii), one *liang*; *Du Zhong* (Cortex Eucommiae Ulmoidis), two *liang*; *Mu Gua* (Fructus Chaenomelis Lagenariae), one *liang*; *Lu Jiao Jiao* (Gelatinum Cornu Cervi), four *liang*, mix-fried with wine; *Hu Gu* (Os Tigridis), two *liang*; mix-fried with vinegar; *Fu Ling* (Sclerotium Poriae Cocos), two *liang*; *Huang Bai* (Cortex Phellodendri), two *liang*, stir-fried with wine; *Chen Pi* (Pericarpium Citri Reticulatae), one *liang*; salt(-processed) *Zhi Mu* (Rhizoma Anemarrhenae Asphodeloidis), two *liang*; *Shu Fu Zi* (Radix Lateralis Praeparatus Aconiti Carmichaeli), five *qian*; *Mai Dong* (Tuber Ophiopogonis Japonici), two *liang*; and *Wu Wei Zi* (Fructus Schisandrae Chinensis), one *liang*. Powder these together make into pills the size of firmiana seeds with heated honey. Take 100 pills each time with wine. It is also alright to take them in the form of a decoction.

*Qing Zao Tang* (Clearing & Drying Decoction)

*Qing Zao* includes *Si Jun* (Four Gentlemen [Decoction]) plus *Cang Zhu* (Rhizoma Atractylodis), *Chen Pi* (Pericarpium Citri Reticulatae), *Huang Qi* (Radix Astragali Membranacei), *Ze Xie* (Rhizoma Alismatis), *Mai Dong* (Tuber Ophiopogonis Japonici), *Dang Gui* (Radix Angelicae Sinensis), *Sheng Ma* (Rhizoma Cimicifugae), *Chai Hu* (Radix Bupleuri), *Huang Lian*

(Rhizoma Coptidis Chinensis), *Wu Wei Zi* (Fructus Schisandrae Chinensis), *Ge Gen* (Radix Puerariae), *Sheng Di* (uncooked Radix Rehmanniae), *Shen Qu* (Massa Medica Fermentata), *Huang Bai* (Cortex Phellodendri), and *Zhu Ling* (Sclerotium Polypori Umbellati). This is a good (formula).

## 52. Impediment Is Caused by Overwhelming Cold, Dampness & Wind

The *Nei Jing (Inner Classic)* says, "The three qi — wind, cold and dampness — may come in a mixed way and join together to produce impediment." If there is mostly wind, this results in migratory (pain). If there is mostly cold, this leads to contracting pain. If there is mostly dampness, this leads to heaviness and fixed (pain). Impediment means block. When wind, cold, and dampness invade the muscles and flesh, they stream along the channels and network vessels. As a result, fluids become unclear, possibly turning into phlegm rheum or produce blood stasis which then obstruct the tunnels and passageways. Therefore, pain arises which may be migratory or there may be numbness and insensitivity. It is appropriate to use *Tong Jing Zhi Tong Tang* (Free the Channels & Stop Pain Decoction).

There was (once) a woman who had been pregnant for two months. She suffered from pain all over her body. The (attending) physician had treated the case as pain wind, but hundreds of medicinals had been ineffective. After nearly one month (of treatment), she did not have one grain (of rice) for several days and her numbness became more serious. (In addition,) she suffered from such serious panting (*i.e.*, asthma) that it nearly killed her. Her pulse was sometimes large and sometimes small. Her face was sometimes red and sometimes white. (I) prescribed one *liang* of *Zuo Chan Teng* (Ramus Lonicerae Japonicae) decocted in two cups of river water. This was administered and recovery ensued in no time.

*Tong Jing Zhi Tong Tang* (Free the Channels & Stop Pain Decoction)

*Tong Jing Zhi Tong Tang* is composed of *Nan Xing* (Rhizoma Arisaematis), *Wei Ling Xian* (Radix Clematidis Chinensis), *Bai Zhi* (Radix Angelicae

Dahuricae), *Huang Bai* (Cortex Phellodendri), *Cang Zhu* (Rhizoma Atractylodis), *Chuan Xiong* (Radix Ligustici Wallichii), *Tao Ren* (Semen Pruni Persicae), *Long Dan Cao* (Radix Gentianae Scabrae), *Shen Qu* (Massa Medica Fermentata), *Fang Ji* (Radix Stephaniae Tetrandrae), *Gui Zhi* (Ramulus Cinnamomi Cassiae), *Hong Hua* (Flos Carthami Tinctorii), and *Qiang Huo* (Radix Et Rhizoma Notopterygii).

## 53. The Four Categories of Seminal Emission Are All Due to Noninteraction of the Heart & Kidneys

Seminal emission has four (types). There is seminal loss due to failure of the heart to control the kidneys as a result of excessive exertion of the heart. There is incessant slippery discharge due to excessive sexual desire. There is essence qi exiting due to its failure to keep to its position as a result of thinking and desire not being followed (*i.e.,* frustration). There is fullness and discharge of essence qi as a result of having no sexual affairs for a long time. All this is ascribed to water and fire not being able to benefit (each other) as a result of the heart and kidneys not connecting (with each other).

Discharge of essence while dreaming of intercourse is called dream emission. This is due to the spirit mind not being clear (and requires) *Er Chen Tang* (Two Aged [Ingredients] Decoction) plus *Ren Shen* (Radix Panacis Ginseng), *Zhi Shi* (Fructus Immaturus Citri Aurantii), *Yuan Zhi* (Radix Polygalae Tenuifoliae), *Fu Shen* (Sclerotium Pararadicis Poriae Cocos), *Suan Zao Ren* (Semen Zizyphi Spinosae), *Chen Sha* (Cinnabar), and *Sha Ren* (Fructus Amomi). Essence exiting with urine is called seminal efflux. This is due to excessive sexual affairs (and requires) *Ba Zhen Tang* (Eight Pearls Decoction) plus *Zhi Mu* (Rhizoma Anemarrhenae Asphodeloidis), *Huang Bai* (Cortex Phellodendri), *Wu Wei Zi* (Fructus Schisandrae Chinensis), *Shan Zhu Yu* (Fructus Corni Officinalis), *Mu Li* (Concha Ostreae), and *Long Gu* (Os Draconis).

A young person (seemingly) had not had sexual intercourse for a long time. He discharged a sticky, slimy thread of essence which often did not even need urination to issue out. I said, "This is seminal efflux (due to) stirring of lust fire making the essence exit." The appropriate treatment was to clear the heart, enrich the kidneys, fortify the spleen, and secure desertion. (I) treated him with *Jiu Long Dan* (Nine Dragons Elixir) and achieved a cure.

*Jiu Long Dan* (Nine Dragons Elixir)

*Jiu Long Dan* is composed of nine flavors: *Jin Ying Zi* (Fructus Rosae Laevigatae), *Shan Zhu Yu* (Fructus Corni Officinalis), *Gou Qi* (Fructus Lycii Chinensis), *Lian Xu* (Stamen Nelumbinis Nuciferae), *Qian Shi* (Semen Euryalis Ferocis), *Fu Ling* (Sclerotium Poriae Cocos), *Shi Lian Zi* (Semen Nelumbinis Nuciferae), *Dang Gui* (Radix Angelicae Sinensis), and *Shu Di* (cooked Radix Rehmanniae).

*Bai Lu Wan* (White Deer Pills)

*Bai Lu* treats seminal emission. It is composed of equal amounts of *Lu Jiao Shuang* (Cornu Degelatinum Cervi) and *Mu Li* (Concha Ostreae) plus a half amount of *Sheng Long Gu* (uncooked Os Draconis). Make these into pills with flour and wine paste and administer.

*Er Chen Tang* (Two Aged [Ingredients] Decoction) [See chapter 11.]

*Ba Zhen Tang* (Eight Pearls Decoction) [See chapter 10.]

## 54. The Five Categories of Jaundice Are Produced by Damp Heat Fuming & Steaming

There are five categories of jaundice, namely, yellow jaundice (*i.e.*, generalized yellowing), yellow sweating, grain jaundice, wine jaundice, and woman (*i.e.*, sexual) taxation jaundice. There are detailed discussions of these in the *Jin Gui Yao Lue* (*Essentials of the Golden Cabinet*). Dan-xi said:

> There is no need to classify jaundice into five categories. All of them are due to damp heat. (The generation of jaundice) is analogous to fermentation.

(To treat jaundice,) first, disinhibit water; second, resolve toxins. The ruling (formula) is *Yin Chen Qu Dan Tang* (Artemisia Capillaris Eliminate Jaundice Decoction). If there is abdominal fullness with a bulging umbilicus and yellowing of the palms and soles of the feet, or if the pulse is absent from the inch opening, jaundice is incurable.

*Yin Chen Qu Dan Tang* (Artemisia Capillaris Eliminate Jaundice Decoction)

*Yin Chen Qu Dan Tang* includes *Huang Qin* (Radix Scutellariae Baicalensis), *Huang Lian* (Rhizoma Coptidis Chinensis), *Zhi Zi* (Fructus Gardeniae Jasminoidis), *Cang Zhu* (Rhizoma Atractylodis), *Zhu Ling* (Sclerotium Polypori Umbellati), *Qing Pi* (Pericarpium Citri Reticulatae Viride), *Ze Xie* (Rhizoma Alismatis), and *Long Dan Cao* (Radix Gentianae Scabrae).[64] Decoct in water and administer.

## 55. Dizziness Never Arises Without Phlegm

The *Ling Shu Jing* (*The Spiritual Pivot Classic*) says:

> The brain is the sea of marrow. When the sea of marrow is superabundant, (the person) is nimble, energetic, and strong and can accomplish what is (normally) beyond one's ability. If the sea of marrow is insufficient, there will be brain spinning, ringing in the ears, aching in the legs, veiling dizziness, loss of vision, fatigue, and somnolence.

Dan-xi said, "Without phlegm there is no dizziness (since) it is phlegm which causes fire to stir." According to my study, dizziness is invariably due to excess of bedroom taxation. When essence is gone, the marrow becomes empty. Then, when taxation (*i.e.*, exertion) stirs, this leads to fire qi flaming upward. As a result, head spinning, eye dimming, and fainting occur. To treat this, it is necessary to greatly supplement the kidneys with *Liu Wei Di Huang Wan* (Six Flavors Rehmannia Pills) plus *Lu Rong* (Cornu

---

[64] Although the text makes no mention of Herba Artemisiae Capillaris (*Yin Chen Hao*) in the list of ingredients, judging from the name of this formula, its inclusion is taken for granted.

Parvum Cervi) and *Niu Xi* (Radix Achyranthis Bidentatae). It is said in the *Nei Jing (Inner Classic)*, "To enrich the sprout one must secure the root (*gen*) and this is the method of treating the root (*ben*)."

If it is phlegm in the chest that causes dizziness and vertigo, the treatment is to use *Er Chen Tang* (Two Aged [Ingredients] Decoction) as the ruling (formula). If mixed with wind, add *Ju Hua* (Flos Chrysanthemi Morifolii), *Tian Ma* (Rhizoma Gastrodiae Elatae), *Chuan Xiong* (Radix Ligustici Wallichii), and *Qiang Huo* (Radix Et Rhizoma Notopterygii). If mixed with cold, add *Fu Zi* (Radix Lateralis Praeparatus Aconiti Carmichaeli) and *Gan Jiang* (dry Rhizoma Zingiberis). If mixed with summerheat, add *Xiang Ru* (Herba Elsholtziae Seu Moslae), *Bian Dou* (Semen Dolichori Lablab), and *Huang Lian* (Rhizoma Coptidis Chinensis). If mixed with dampness, add *Cang Zhu* (Rhizoma Atractylodis), *Bai Zhu* (Rhizoma Atractylodis Macrocephalae), and *Gan Jiang* (dry Rhizoma Zingiberis).

If a (sick) person suffers from dizziness due to blood desertion as a result of excessive ejection of blood, flooding, or delivery, it is appropriate to supplement (the blood) with *Du Shen Tang* (Solitary Ginseng Decoction). This is the method of boosting the qi (to treat) blood collapse.

*Liu Wei Di Huang Wan* (Six Flavors Rehmannia Pills)

*Liu Wei Di Huang Wan* are composed of decocted *Dan Pi* (Cortex Radicis Moutan) and *Shan Yao* (Radix Dioscoreae Oppositae) and *Shan Zhu Yu* (Fructus Corni Officinalis), *Fu Ling* (Sclerotium Poriae Cocos), *Ze Xie* (Rhizoma Alismatis), and *Shu Di* (cooked Radix Rehmanniae) made into pills.

*Er Chen Tang* (Two Aged [Ingredients] Decoction) [See chapter 11.]

# 56. Wasting Thirst Never Arises Without Fire

There are three categories of wasting thirst. Upper wasting is ascribed to the lungs. (It manifests) as polydipsia and reduced eating with normal urination and defecation. Middle wasting is ascribed to the stomach. (It manifests) as polyphagia with rapid hungering and yellow or reddish urine. Lower wasting is ascribed to the kidneys. (It manifests) as strangury of turbid, unctuous urine, vexatious thirst with polydipsia, black, parched helix, and frequent urination (*i.e.*, polyuria). If there is ability to eat, there is bound to be welling abscesses, flat abscesses, and sores on the back. If there is inability to eat, there is bound to be transformation of center fullness and abdominal distention.

Generally speaking, the three categories of wasting are all due to the heat qi of fire stewing the viscera and bowels and consuming the blood. Their treatment is to use *Si Wu Tang* (Four Materials Decoction) as the ruling (formula). For upper wasting, add *Ren Shen* (Radix Panacis Ginseng), *Wu Wei Zi* (Fructus Schisandrae Chinensis), *Mai Dong* (Tuber Ophiopogonis Japonici), and *Hua Fen* (Radix Trichosanthis Kirlowii). Decoct these and then put in *Ou Zhi* (Succus Rhizomatis Nelumbinis Nuciferae), *Ren Ru* (Lac Hominis), and *Sheng Di Zhi* (uncooked Radix Rehmanniae juice). For alcoholics, add uncooked *Ge Gen Zhi* (Radix Puerariae juice). For middle wasting, add *Shi Gao* (Gypsum Fibrosum) to downbear stomach fire. For lower wasting, add *Huang Bai* (Cortex Phellodendri), *Zhi Mu* (Rhizoma Anemarrhenae Asphodeloidis), and *Wu Wei Zi* (Fructus Schisandrae Chinensis) to enrich kidney water.

*Si Wu Tang* (Four Materials Decoction) [See chapter 10.]

# 57. Insomnia Is Due to Phlegm Fire Effulgence & Shortage of Blood

Insomnia has three (categories). There is insomnia due to the spirit failing to return to its abode as a result of existence of phlegm in the heart channel. (To treat this,) prescribe *Wen Dan Tang* (Warm the Gallbladder Decoction) plus *Suan Zao Ren* (Semen Zizyphi Spinosae), *Zhu Li* (Succus Bambusae), and *Jiang Zhi* (Succus Rhizomatis Zingiberis). There is insomnia due to vacuity weakness following disease. (To treat this,) use *Liu Jun Tang* (Six Gentlemen Decoction) plus *Huang Qi* (Radix Astragali Membranacei) and *Suan Zao Ren* (Semen Zizyphi Spinosae). There is insomnia due to shortage of blood (which requires) *Gui Pi Tang* (Return the Spleen Decoction). In addition, insomnia may be due to gallbladder vacuity cold. (To treat this,) grind stir-fried *Zao Ren* (Semen Zizyphi Spinosae) into powder and take with *Zhu Ye* (Folium Bambusae) soup. Profuse sleeping may be due to gallbladder replete heat.[65] (To treat this,) grind uncooked *Suan Zao Ren* (Semen Zizyphi Spinosae) into powder and take with ginger and tea soup.

*Wen Dan Tang* (Warm the Gallbladder Decoction) [See chapter 11.]

*Liu Jun Tang* (Six Gentlemen Decoction) [See chapter 9.]

*Gui Pi Tang* (Return the Spleen Decoction) [See #40 above.]

## 58. Profuse Sleeping Is Due to Spleen-Stomach Fatigue & Spirit Clouding

When the spleen and stomach are fatigued, listlessness and somnolence will arise. If there is shortage of spirit, laziness and profuse sleeping will arise. *Liu Jun Tang* (Six Gentlemen Decoction) is the ruling formula (for these conditions).

## 59. Constipation Is Due to Blood & Fluid Dryness & Binding

Constipation is a result of desiccation of fluids and humors. To treat this, it is necessary to nourish the blood and moisten the intestines. The appropriate (formula) is *Si Wu Tang* (Four Materials Decoction) plus *Ma Ren* (Semen Cannabis Sativae), *Xing Ren* (Semen Pruni Armeniacae), etc. One should not frenetically (*i.e.*, recklessly) use drastic precipitating medicinals like *Mang Xiao* (Mirabilitum), *Da Huang* (Radix Et Rhizoma

---

[65] The translator suspects there is a typographical error here and that this line should read insomnia rather than profuse sleeping. *Suan Zao Ren* (Semen Zizyphi Spinosae) is a famous medicinal for insomnia and does not supplement the qi or yang, while gallbladder replete heat should only cause stirring and restlessness, not somnolence.

Rhei), *Ba Dou* (Semen Crotinis Tiglii), and *Qian Niu* (Semen Pharbiditis). These fell and cause detriment to true yin and vanquish and damage the stomach qi. Contrarily, they result in great harm (rather than any good). If the stomach qi is replete with evils lodged within the intestines, there is no other choice but to apply precipitation. Then the use of medicinals like *Mang Xiao* (Mirabilitum) and *Da Huang* (Radix Et Rhizoma Rhei) is necessary.

*Run Zao Tang* (Moisten Dryness Decoction)

*Run Zao Tang* is composed of nine flavors: *Tao Ren* (Semen Pruni Persicae), *Hong Hua* (Flos Carthami Tinctorii), *Dang Gui* (Radix Angelicae Sinensis), *Sheng Di* (uncooked Radix Rehmanniae), *Shu Di* (cooked Radix Rehmanniae), *Gan Cao* (Radix Glycyrrhizae), *Da Huang* (Radix Et Rhizoma Rhei), *Ma Ren* (Semen Cannabis Sativae), and *Sheng Ma* (Rhizoma Cimicifugae).

# 60. Urinary Block Is Due to Stagnant Qi Not Moving

Dong-yuan said, "Urinary stoppage is classified by thirst and absence of thirst, and its treatment differs depending upon (heat) lodging in the qi or blood divisions." If inhibited urination is accompanied by thirst, evils are located in the qi division of the upper burner. This requires clearing the lung qi and draining fire to enrich the upper source of water. The ruling (formula) is *Qing Fei Yin* (Clear the Lungs Drink). If inhibited urination is accompanied by absence of thirst, heat is in the blood division of the lower burner. This requires eliminating heat evils to enrich the lower source of water of the urinary bladder and kidneys. The ruling (formula) is *Tong Guan Wan* (Free the Pass Pills).

A person (once) suffered from non-free flowing urination. Administration of various medicinals had been ineffective. I said, "The urinary bladder holds the office of the river islands and stores fluids and humors. When qi transforms, (fluids) are able to exit. Now urination is not freely flowing. This is because qi is stagnant." (I) stir-fried *Da Zao Jiao* (Fructus Gleditschiae Chinensis) till scorched, ground this into powder, and made this into pills with honey the size of firmiana seeds. (The patient) took these with boiled water. Seven pills effected recovery.

*Qing Fei Yin* (Clear the Lungs Drink)

*Qing Fei Yin* (is composed of) *Zhu Ling* (Sclerotium Polypori Umbellati), *Ze Xie* (Rhizoma Alismatis), *Mu Tong* (Caulis Akebiae), *Che Qian Zi* (Semen Plantaginis), *Tong Cao* (Medulla Tetrapanacis Papyriferi) *Qu Mai* (Herba Dianthi), *Deng Xin* (Medulla Junci Effusi), *Bian Xu* (Herba Polygoni Avicularis), and *Fu Ling* (Sclerotium Poriae Cocos). Decoct and mix with powdered *Hu Po* (Succinum).

*Tong Guan Wan* (Free the Pass Pills) [a.k.a. *Zi Shen Wan*, Enrich the Kidneys Pills]

*Tong Guan Wan* (are composed of) *Zhi Mu* (Rhizoma Anemarrhenae Asphodeloidis) and *Huang Bai* (Cortex Phellodendri), two *lian* each, mix-fried with wine, and *Rou Gui* (Cortex Cinnamomi Cassiae), one *qian*. Take these with water on an empty stomach.

# 61. Hemorrhoidal Disease & Intestinal Wind Are the Result of Damp Heat

Hemorrhoidal disease is ruled by the qi of damp heat. Like fungi growing on a tree, (hemorrhoids) are invariably the product of damp heat. (Therefore,) their treatment should cool the blood and loosen the qi as the ruling (method). I have designed a formula using *Tiao Qin* (young Radix Scutellariae Baicalensis), *Huang Lian* (Rhizoma Coptidis Chinensis), *Qin Jiao* (Radix Gentianae Macrophyllae), *Dang Gui* (Radix Angelicae Sinensis), *Sheng Di* (cooked Radix Rehmanniae), *Jing Jie* (Herba Schizonepetae Tenuifoliae), *Fang Feng* (Radix Ledebouriellae Divaricatae), *Gan Cao* (Radix Glycyrrhizae), *Qing Pi* (Pericarpium Citri Reticulatae Viride), *Zhi Ke* (Fructus Citri Aurantii), *Huai Jiao* (Fructus Sophorae Japonicae), and *Bai Zhu* (Rhizoma Atractylodis Macrocephalae). Decoct these in water and administer. Externally, grind three *li* of *Bing Pian* (Borneol), three *fen* of male pig's gall [better bear's gall], and one piece of *Fan Mu Bie* (Semen

Strychnotis) in well water into a thick solution. Then apply it. Relief will occur that very day. I have had many (successful) experiences with this treatment.

Blood in the stools: If (the blood) is clear and fresh colored, this is called intestinal wind. If (the blood) is turbid and black colored, this is called visceral toxins. Bleeding preceding stools is known as near bleeding. Bleeding at the end of defecation is known as far bleeding. For both, use *Dang Gui He Xue San* (Dang Gui Harmonize the Blood Powder).

*Dang Gui He Xue San* (Dang Gui Harmonize the Blood Powder)

*Dang Gui He Xue San* (includes) *Chuan Xiong* (Radix Ligustici Wallichii), *Bai Zhu* (Rhizoma Atractylodis Macrocephalae), *Sheng Ma* (Rhizoma Cimicifugae), *Huai Hua* (Flos Immaturus Sophorae Japonicae), *Qing Pi* (Pericarpium Citri Reticulatae Viride), *Jing Jie* (Herba Schizonepetae Tenuifoliae), and *Shu Di* (cooked Radix Rehmanniae). It can lighten (*i.e.*, relieve) the disease of intestinal wind.

*Wu Mei Wan* (Mume Pills)

Burn *Wu Mei* (Fructus Pruni Mume) to charcoal, grind, and make into pills with flour and vinegar paste. Take with rice soup on an empty stomach. This can cure hemafecia instantly.

# 62. Macular Eruptions & Addictive Papules Are Produced by Overwhelming Wind Heat

Macular eruptions (refer to) the outbreak of cloud-shaped red patches on the skin. Addictive papules are spots on the skin like flea bites in form. Both are due to overwhelming wind heat. To treat them, use *Xi Jiao Xiao Du Yin* (Rhinoceros Horn Disperse Toxins Beverage). If there is constipation, *Fang Feng Tong Sheng San* (Ledebouriella Sage-communicated Powder) is the ruling (formula).

*Xi Jiao Xiao Du Yin* (Rhinoceros Horn Disperse Toxins Beverage)

*Xi Jiao Xiao Du Yin* (includes) *Niu Bang Zi* (Fructus Arctii Lappae), *Fang Feng* (Radix Ledebouriellae Divaricatae), *Jing Jie* (Herba Schizonepetae Tenuifoliae), and *Gan Cao* (Radix Glycyrrhizae). It can eliminate red patches in a minute.

*Fang Feng Tong Sheng San* (Ledebouriella Sage-communicated Powder) [See #7 above.]

# 63. Deafness Is a Result of Kidney Vacuity

The ears are the orifices of the kidneys. If the kidney qi is replete, the ears can hear. If the kidney qi is vacuous, the ears will be deaf. This is a great (*i.e.*, general or rough) analysis. In fact, since (the ears) are on the routes of the two channels of the hand *shao yang* of the triple burner and foot *shao yang* of the gallbladder, there may be qi reversal deafness, deafness mixed with wind, and taxation damage deafness which must be treated according to the condition (*i.e.*, each one differently). Kidney vacuity deafness (requires) *Si Wu Tang* (Four Materials Decoction) plus *Gou Qi* (Fructus Lycii Chinensis), *Cong Rong* (Herba Cistanchis Deserticolae), *Zhi Mu* (Rhizoma Anemarrhenae Asphodeloidis), *Huang Bai* (Cortex Phellodendri), *Chang Pu* (Rhizoma Acori Graminei), and *Chai Hu* (Radix Bupleuri). Qi deafness (requires) *Er Chen Tang* (Two Aged [Ingredients] Decoction) plus *Xiang Fu* (Rhizoma Cyperi Rotundi), *Mu Xiang* (Radix Auklandiae Lappae), *Huang Qin* (Radix Scutellariae Baicalensis), *Long Dan Cao* (Radix Gentianae Scabrae), *Chai Hu* (Radix Bupleuri), and *Chang Pu* (Rhizoma Acori Graminei). Wind deafness (requires) *Jiu Wei Qiang Huo Tang* (Nine Flavors Notopterygium Decoction) plus *Chai Hu* (Radix Bupleuri) and *Chang Pu* (Rhizoma Acori Graminei). (And) taxation deafness (requires) *Bu Zhong Yi Qi Tang* (Supplement the Center & Boost the Qi Decoction) plus *Yuan Zhi* (Radix Polygalae Tenuifoliae) and *Chang Pu* (Rhizoma Acori Graminei).

*Si Wu Tang* (Four Materials Decoction) [See chapter 10.]

*Er Chen Tang* (Two Aged [Ingredients] Decoction) [See chapter 11.]

*Jiu Wei Qiang Huo Tang* (Nine Flavors Notopterygium Decoction) [See #4 above.]

*Bu Zhong Yi Qi Tang* (Supplement the Center & Boost the Qi Decoction) [See #5, above.]

# 64. The Cause of Eye Disease Is Liver Fire

Zhang Zi-he said, "The eyes are the external manifestation of the liver." He also said:

> Although (past) sages have said that, so long as the eyes are supplied with blood, they can see, (however,) blood may be superabundant or insufficient. Superabundance produces congestion and pain in the eyes, while insufficiency causes exhaustion and, hence, loss of vision of the eyes. Generally speaking, young people are liable to suffer from superabundance, while old, [thin, and weak] people from insufficiency.

The great (treatment) method is drainage in case of repletion and supplementationase of vacuity. The method of prescription to treat eye (disease is as follows). To dissipate wind, use *Fang Feng* (Radix Ledebouriellae Divaricatae), *Jing Jie* (Herba Schizonepetae Tenuifoliae), *Qiang Huo* (Radix Et Rhizoma Notopterygii), *Bai Zhi* (Radix Angelicae Dahuricae), *Man Jing Zi* (Fructus Viticis), *Ju Hua* (Flos Chrysanthemi Morifolii), *Bo He* (Herba Menthae Haplocalysis), and the like. To clear heat, use *Huang Qin* (Radix Scutellariae Baicalensis), *Huang Lian* (Rhizoma Coptidis Chinensis), *Zhi Zi* (Fructus Gardeniae Jasminoidis), *Huang Bai* (Cortex Phellodendri), *Lian Qiao* (Fructus Forsythiae Suspensae), *Zhi Mu* (Rhizoma Anemarrhenae Asphodeloidis), *Dan Cao* (Radix Gentianae Scabrae), and the like. To nourish the blood, use *Dang Gui* (Radix Angelicae Sinensis), *Chuan Xiong* (Radix Ligustici Wallichii), *Bai Shao* (Radix Albus Paeoniae Lactiflorae), *Sheng Di* (uncooked Radix Rehmanniae), *Shu Di* (cooked Radix Rehmanniae), *Gou Qi* (Fructus Lycii

Chinensis), *Xia Ku Cao* (Spica Prunellae Vulgaris), and the like. To rectify the qi, use *Xiang Fu* (Rhizoma Cyperi Rotundi), *Zhi Ke* (Fructus Citri Aurantii), *Qing Pi* (Pericarpium Citri Reticulatae Viride), *Bing Lang* (Semen Arecae Catechu), *Bai Dou Kou* (Fructus Cardamomi), *Cang Zhu* (Rhizoma Atractylodis), *Gan Cao* (Radix Glycyrrhizae), and the like. To supplement the qi, use *Ren Shen* (Radix Panacis Ginseng), *Huang Qi* (Radix Astragali Membranacei), *Bai Zhu* (Rhizoma Atractylodis Macrocephalae), and the like. To eliminate eye screen, use *Mu Zei* (Herba Equiseti Hiemalis), *Ji Li* (Fructus Tribuli Terrestris), *Chan Tui* (Periostracum Cicadae), *She Tui* (Exuviae Serpentis), and the like. To brighten the eyes, use *Mi Meng Hua* (Flos Buddleiae Officinalis), *Gu Jing Cao* (Scapus Et Inflorescentia Eriocaulonis Buergeriani), *Qing Xiang Zi* (Semen Celosiae Argenteae), *Cao Jue Ming* (Semen Cassiae Torae), *Yang Gan* (goat liver), *Chai Hu* (Radix Bupleuri), and the like.

## 65. Toothache Is a Result of Stomach Heat & Qi Vacuity

The teeth are the ends of the kidneys and the surplus of the bones. If the kidneys are replete, the teeth are secure. If the kidneys are vacuous, the teeth are loose. Toothache, (however,) is not concerned with the kidneys but is due to the heat in the *yang ming* channels. It should be treated with *Qing Wei San* (Clear the Stomach Powder). If qi vacuity is the cause of pain, prescribe *Bu Zhong Yi Qi Tang* (Supplement the Center & Boost the Qi Decoction) plus *Shu Di* (cooked Radix Rehmanniae), *Dan Pi* (Cortex Radicis Moutan), *Fu Ling* (Sclerotium Poriae Cocos), and *Bai Shao* (Radix Albus Paeoniae Lactiflorae). If there is a hole (*i.e.*, a cavity), powder *Chuan Jiao* (Pericarpium Zanthoxyli Bungeani) and *Shao Shi Hui* (Slaked Lime), make into pills with honey, and fill in the hole. Then relief will ensue. For *gan* of the teeth and gums[66], burn *Wu Bei Zi* (Galla Rhois Chinensis) to ash, mix with a small amount of powdered *Long Gu* (Os Draconis), and dab (the *gan*). This is miraculously effective.

---

[66] This refers to erythematous swelling and ulceration of the gums.

*Qing Wei San* (Clear the Stomach Powder)

*Qing Wei San* uses *Sheng Ma* (Rhizoma Cimicifugae), *Huang Lian* (Rhizoma Coptidis Chinensis), *Dang Gui* (Radix Angelicae Sinensis), *Sheng Di* (uncooked Radix Rehmanniae), and *Mu Dan Pi* (Cortex Radicis Moutan). *Shi Gao* (Gypsum Fibrosum) may be added. This calms stomach heat and is appropriate for mouth sores, ejection (of blood), nosebleeding, and gaping gums.

# 66. Throat Impediment Is Due to Stirring Fire & Upborne Phlegm

Throat impediment is congestion and non-free flow of the throat. It may (also) be called nipple moth and throat-entwining wind. Although it has various names, its causes are but fire and phlegm. If the pulse is floating and faint, it is incurable. The method of using medicinals (is as follows). To clear heat, use *Huang Lian* (Rhizoma Coptidis Chinensis), *Yuan Shen* (Radix Scrophulariae Ningpoensis), *Shan Dou Gen* (Radix Sophorae Subprostratae), and *Deng Xin* (Medulla Junci Effusi). To resolve toxins, use *She Gan* (Rhizoma Belamcandae Chinensis), *Niu Bang Zi* (Fructus Arctii Lappae), and *Gan Cao* (Radix Glycyrrhizae). To disperse phlegm, use *Bei Mu* (Bulbus Fritillariae), *Hua Fen* (Radix Trichosanthis Kirlowii), *Fu Ling* (Sclerotium Poriae Cocos), *Jie Geng* (Radix Platycodi Grandiflori), and *Zhi Ke* (Fructus Citri Aurantii). To enrich yin, use *Bai Shao* (Radix Albus Paeoniae Lactiflorae), *Sheng Di* (uncooked Radix Rehmanniae), *Huang Bai* (Cortex Phellodendri), *Zhi Mu* (Rhizoma Anemarrhenae Asphodeloidis), and *Zhu Li* (Succus Bambusae)

A young person returned from a long trip on a fiercely hot day and was subsequently taken with sudden congestion and block of the throat with a red facial complexion and tearing. Determining that sudden disease is ascribed to fire and that odd diseases are ascribed to phlegm, I powdered five *fen* of *Chen Sha* (Cinnabar) and two *qian* of *Bai Fan* (Alum), mixing them with cold water, and administered them. Cure ensued in no time. In addition, I (once) treated a phlegm condition with loss of voice. When the medicinals were taken, the ability to speak was restored. The formula was the same as above.

# 67. Nasal Congestion Is Due to Inhibited Lung Qi

The nose is the orifice of the lungs. There are two patterns of nasal congestion. (First,) nasal congestion is accompanied by inability to detect fragrance from fetor. It may happen once the cold months come or occur as a result of contraction of the slightest wind cold. In (the former) case, there have been fire evils in the lung channel. When fire becomes severe, a liking for heat and aversion to cold will arise. Therefore, in winter nasal congestion will never fail to occur and, when (the nose is) exposed to wind, it never fails to arise. (Secondly,) nasal congestion with heavy voice occasionally may (also) happen as a result of contraction of wind cold (in any season). This should be naturally treated as wind cold. Generally speaking, diseases of the nose, except for wind damage nasal congestion, are invariably caused by fire heat and require using heat-clearing medicinals.

*Xin Yi San* (Magnolia Flower Powder)

*Xin Yi San* includes *Gao Ben* (Radix Et Rhizoma Ligustici Chinensis), *Fang Feng* (Radix Ledebouriellae Divaricatae), *Bai Zhi* (Radix Angelicae Dahuricae), *Sheng Ma* (Rhizoma Cimicifugae), *Mu Tong* (Xaulis Akebiae), *Chuan Xiong* (Radix Ligustici Wallichii), *Xi Xin* (Herba Asari Cum Radice), and *Gan Cao* (Radix Glycyrrhizae). Take these mixed with tea. This formula is (also) used to cure nasal polyps.

*Cang Er San* (Xanthium Powder)

In *Cang Er San*, four flavors are used, including *Bo He* (Herba Menthae Haplocalysis), *Xin Yi* (Flos Magnoliae Liliflorae), and *Bai Zhi* (Radix Angelicae Dahuricae). These are taken mixed with scallion and tea. It courses the liver and lungs, upbears the clear and downbears the turbid. (It cures) deep-source nasal congestion.

# 68. Mouth Sores Are Due to Wandering Spleen Fire

The mouth is the external manifestation of the spleen. When spleen fire goes upward, sores will grow in the mouth. To treat this, (administer) *Xie Huang San* (Drain the Yellow Powder) and (externally) apply powdered *Huang Lian* (Rhizoma Coptidis Chinensis) and *Gan Jiang* (dry Rhizoma Zingiberis). In case of vacuity fire flaming upward, if cool medicinals fail to bring effect, treat this with *Li Zhong Tang* (Rectify the Center Decoction). When there is heat in the heart, there will be a bitter taste in the mouth. Treat this with *Xie Xin Tang* (Drain the Heart Decoction). If there is heat in the spleen, there will be a sweet taste in the mouth. Treat this with *Xie Huang San* (Drain the Yellow Powder). When there is heat in the lungs, there will be a peppery taste in the mouth. Treat this with *Xie Bai San* (Drain the White Powder). If there is heat in the kidneys, there will be a salty taste in the mouth. Treat this with *Zi Shen Wan* (Enrich the Kidneys Pills). When there is replete heat in the liver and gallbladder, there will be a sour and bitter taste in the mouth and the appropriate (medicinals) are *Chai Hu* (Radix Bupleuri), *Long Dan Cao* (Radix Gentianae Scabrae), *Qing Pi* (Pericarpium Citri Reticulatae Viride), *Huang Qin* (Radix Scutellariae Baicalensis), and the like. If there is vacuity heat in the stomach, there will be a bland taste in the mouth. This requires *Bu Zhong Yi Qi Tang* (Supplement the Center & Boost the Qi Decoction). If dry, cracked lips are accompanied by (mouth) sores, there is insufficiency of spleen blood. This requires *Gui Pi Tang* (Return the Spleen Decoction).

*Xie Huang San* (Drain the Yellow Powder)

*Xie Huang* (is composed of) *Gan Cao* (Radix Glycyrrhizae), *Fang Feng* (Radix Ledebouriellae Divaricatae), *Shi Gao* (Gypsum Fibrosum), *Zhi Zi* (Fructus Gardeniae Jasminoidis), and *Huo Xiang* (Herba Agastachis Seu Pogostemi). Stir-fry these with honey and wine till fragrant and then administer. This (formula) is effective when stomach fire and mouth sores are seen together.

*Xie Bai San* (Drain the White Powder)

*Xie Bai* (is composed of) four ingredients: *Sang Pi* (Cortex Radicis Mori Albi), *Di Gu Pi* (Cortex Radicis Lycii Chinensis), *Gan Cao* (Radix Glycyrrhizae), and *Jing Mi* (Semen Oryzae Sativae). (However,) it may also include *Ren Shen* (Radix Panacis Ginseng), *Fu Ling* (Sclerotium Poriae Cocos), *Zhi Mu* (Rhizoma Anemarrhenae Asphodeloidis), and *Huang Qin* (Radix Scutellariae Baicalensis). This may (also) be administered when there is lung heat panting and coughing.

*Zi Shen Wan* (Enrich the Kidneys Pills) [*i.e., Tong Guan Wan,* Free the Pass Pills] [See #50 above.]

*Li Zhong Tang* (Rectify the Center Decoction) [See #3 above.]

*Xie Xin Tang* (Drain the Heart Decoction) [See #3 above.]

*Bu Zhong Yi Qi Tang* (Supplement the Center & Boost the Qi Decoction) [See #5 above.]

*Gui Pi Tang* (Return the Spleen Decoction) [See #40 above.]

# 69. Women's Menstrual Irregularities Are All Ascribed to Qi Counterflow

Dan-xi's discussion of the menses can be summarized (as follows). Menstrual water is yin blood. The blood is the spouse of the qi and relies on the qi for its movement. Clots in the menstrual flow are produced by qi congelation. Pain arising as the menses move (*i.e.,* premenstrually and at their onset) is due to qi stagnation. Postmenstrual pain is due to vacuity of both qi and blood. Pale (menstrual flow) is due to profuse phlegm and also vacuity. Crossed menstruation[67] (due to) frenetic movement (of

---

[67] Crossed menstruation refers to vicarious menstruation, *i.e.,* bleeding at the time of menstruation either or simultaneously from some other orifice than the vagina.

blood) is caused by chaotic qi. Purple (menstrual flow) is due to qi heat. If it is black, the heat is severe. For all categories of menstrual irregularity, one should prescribe *Si Wu Tang* (Four Materials Decoction) as the ruling (formula).

The method of using medicinals (are as follows). To supplement the qi, use *Ren Shen* (Radix Panacis Ginseng), *Bai Zhu* (Rhizoma Atractylodis Macrocephalae), *Huang Qi* (Radix Astragali Membranacei), and *Gan Cao* (Radix Glycyrrhizae). To supplement the blood, use *Dang Gui* (Radix Angelicae Sinensis), *Chuan Xiong* (Radix Ligustici Wallichii), *Bai Shao* (Radix Albus Paeoniae Lactiflorae), *Shu Di* (cooked Radix Rehmanniae), *Ai Ye* (Folium Artemisiae Argyi), *E Jiao* (Gelatinum Corii Asini), and carbonized *Pu Huang* (Pollen Typhae). For qi stagnation, use *Chen Pi* (Pericarpium Citri Reticulatae), *Xiang Fu* (Rhizoma Cyperi Rotundi), *Wu Yao* (Radix Linderae Strychnifoliae), *E Zhu* (Rhizoma Curcumae Zedoariae), *Qing Pi* (Pericarpium Citri Reticulatae Viride), *Zhi Ke* (Fructus Citri Aurantii), and *Sha Ren* (Fructus Amomi). For blood stagnation, use *Hong Hua* (Flos Carthami Tinctorii), *Tao Ren* (Semen Pruni Persicae), *Gui Wei* (Apex Radicis Angelicae Sinensis), *Dan Pi* (Cortex Radicis Moutan), and *Niu Xi* (Radix Achyranthis Bidentatae). To clear heat, use *Chai Hu* (Radix Bupleuri), *Huang Qin* (Radix Scutellariae Baicalensis), *Zhi Mu* (Rhizoma Anemarrhenae Asphodeloidis), *Huang Bai* (Cortex Phello-dendri), *Huang Lian* (Rhizoma Coptidis Chinensis), and *Sheng Di* (uncooked Radix Rehmanniae). To warm the channels (or menses), use *Gan Jiang* (dry Rhizoma Zingiberis), *Fu Zi* (Radix Lateralis Praeparatus Aconiti Carmichaeli), and *Rou Gui* (Cortex Cinnamomi Cassiae). To relieve pain, use *Sha Ren* (Fructus Amomi) and *Yuan Hu* (Rhizoma Corydalis Yanhusuo). To eliminate phlegm, use *Nan Xing* (Rhizoma Arisaematis) and *Ban Xia* (Rhizoma Pinelliae Ternatae). To stop (bleeding) and astringe, use *Chi Shi Zhi* (Hallyositum Rubrum) and *Fu Long Gan* (Terra Falva Ustae).

*Si Wu Tang* (Four Materials Decoction) [See chapter 10.]

# 70. Women's Heart Vexation & Tidal Fever Mostly Arise From Depression

Women are liable to have depression disease with sometimes chills and sometimes fever, decreased food intake, and an emaciated body. The appropriate (formula) to use is *Yue Ju Wan* (Out-thrust Tribulation Pills) to open depression, and *Xiao Yao San* (Rambling Powder) to regulate the menses.

*Yue Ju Wan* (Out-thrust Tribulation Pills) [See #14, above.]

*Xiao Yao San* (Rambling Powder)

*Xiao Yao San* uses *Dang Gui* (Radix Angelicae Sinensis), *Shao Yao* (Radix Paeoniae Lactiflorae), *Chai Hu* (Radix Bupleuri), *Fu Ling* (Sclerotium Poriae Cocos), *Bai Zhu* (Rhizoma Atractylodis Macrocephalae), *Gan Cao* (Radix Glycyrrhizae), and *Bo He* (Herba Menthae Haplocalysis). It dissipates depression and regulates menstruation with most rapid results. To (specifically) regulate menstruation, (however,) it should be combined with *Dan Pi* (Cortex Radicis Moutan) and *Zhi Zi* (Fructus Gardeniae Jasminoidis).

# 71. The Cause of Vaginal Discharge & Sand Strangury Is Damp Heat

Vaginal discharge looks like snivel, thick and sticky. To treat it, it is necessary to clear the heart and supplement and nourish as the ruling (methods). Sand strangury (is voiding of urine) which is pale and thin like water. To treat it, it is necessary to clear heat and dry dampness as the ruling (methods). If a woman suffers from no disease (otherwise) but has white vaginal discharge, this is due to damp heat streaming down. If a woman suffers from red and white vaginal discharge in an enduring disease, this is due to vacuous qi sunken below. To treat it, use *Gui Pi Tang* (Return the Spleen Decoction) and *Bu Zhong Yi Qi Tang* (Supplement the Center & Boost the Qi Decoction).

A 50 year-old woman suffered from white sand strangury with simultaneous chest and diaphragm constriction. I prescribed *Yue Ju Wan* (Outthrust Tribulation Pills). One dose cured both conditions.

*Yue Ju Wan* (Out-thrust Tribulation Pills) [See #14 above.]

*Gui Pi Tang* (Return the Spleen Decoction) [See #40 above.]

*Bu Zhong Yi Qi Tang* (Supplement the Center & Boost the Qi Decoction) [See #5 above.]

# 72. Flooding & Leaking of Blood Are Due to Detriment of the *Ren* & *Chong*

The disease of flooding and leaking is due to detriment of the *chong* and *ren* vessels. The *chong mai* is the sea of blood of the twelve channels, and the *ren mai* is the original qi of engenderment and nourishment. If these two vessels suffer detriment, the blood will consequently move frenetically. At its onset, (this disease) is categorized as replete heat, requiring clearing heat. Later on, it is categorized as vacuity heat, requiring nourishing the blood and clearing heat. If it endures for (many) days, it is categorized as vacuity cold, requiring warming the channels and supplementing the blood.

To clear heat, (use) *Huang Qin* (Radix Scutellariae Baicalensis), *Huang Lian* (Rhizoma Coptidis Chinensis), *Huang Bai* (Cortex Phellodendri), *Zhi Mu* (Rhizoma Anemarrhenae Asphodeloidis), *Sheng Di* (uncooked Radix Rehmanniae), and *Mai Dong* (Tuber Ophiopogonis Japonici). To supplement the blood, (use) *Dang Gui* (Radix Angelicae Sinensis), *Chuan Xiong* (Radix Ligustici Wallichii), *Bai Shao Yao* (Radix Albus Paeoniae Lactiflorae), *Shu Di* (cooked Radix Rehmanniae), *Ai Ye* (Folium Artemisiae Argyi), *E Jiao* (Gelatinum Corii Asini), and carbonized *Pu Huang* (Pollen Typhae). To supplement the qi, (use) *Ren Shen* (Radix Panacis Ginseng), *Huang Qi* (Radix Astragali Membranacei), *Gan Cao* (Radix Glycyrrhizae), and *Bai Zhu* (Rhizoma Atractylodis Macrocephalae). To regulate the qi, (use) *Chen Pi* (Pericarpium Citri Reticulatae), *Xiang Fu* (Rhizoma Cyperi

Rotundi), and *Sha Ren* (Fructus Amomi). To upbear yang, (use) *Qiang Huo* (Radix Et Rhizoma Notopterygii), *Du Huo* (Radix Angelicae Pubescentis), *Fang Feng* (Radix Ledebouriellae Divaricatae), *Sheng Ma* (Rhizoma Cimicifugae), and *Chai Hu* (Radix Bupleuri). (And) to stop (bleeding) and astringe, (use) *Chi Shi Zhi* (Hallyositum Rubrum) and *Fu Long Gan* (Terra Falva Ustae).

# 73. The Treatment of Disquiet Fetus Has Two Principles

There are two methods for quieting the fetus. If the pregnant woman is diseased and the fetal qi consequently becomes disquieted, only treat the mother's disease and the fetus will become quiet on its own. If the fetal qi is disquieted and this results in the pregnant woman becoming diseased, only quiet the fetal qi and the (mother's) disease will heal on its own.

*Jiao Ai Si Wu Tang* (Gelatin & Mugwort Four Materials Decoction)

*Jiao Ai Tang* is for (fetal) leaking. (It includes) *Chuan Xiong* (Radix Ligustici Wallichii), *Shao Yao* (Radix Paeoniae Lactiflorae), *Dang Gui* (Radix Angelicae Sinensis), *Di Huang* (Radix Rehmanniae), and *Gan Cao* (Radix Glycyrrhizae). It quiets stirring fetus in no time.

*Zi Su Yin* (Perilla Drink)

*Zi Su Yin* is for fetal suspension.[68] (It includes) *Chuan Xiong* (Radix Ligustici Wallichii), *Dang Gui* (Radix Angelicae Sinensis), *Shao Yao* (Radix Paeoniae Lactiflorae), *Chen Pi* (Pericarpium Citri Reticulatae), *Fu Pi* (Pericarpium Arecae Catechu), *Ren Shen* (Radix Panacis Ginseng), and *Gan Cao* (Radix Glycyrrhizae). It instantly relieves distention and fullness.

*Zi Lin San* (Fetal Strangury Powder)

---

[68] Distention and fullness of the chest in pregnancy is called fetal suspension.

*Zi Lin San* (is composed of) *Mai Dong* (Tuber Ophiopogonis Japonici), *Zhu Ye* (Folium Bambusae), *Fu Pi* (Pericarpium Arecae Catechu), *Chi Fu Ling* (Sclerotium Rubrus Poriae Cocos), *Deng Xi* (Medulla Junci Effusi), *Mu Tong* (Caulis Akebiae), and *Gan Cao* (Radix Glycyrrhizae). It instantly resolves difficult urination.

*Ling Yang Jiao San* (Antelope Horn Powder)

For fetal epilepsy[69], drink *Ling Yang* (Cornu Antelopis Saiga-tatarici), *Chuan Xiong* (Radix Ligustici Wallichii), *Dang Gui* (Radix Angelicae Sinensis), *Yi Mi* (Semen Coicis Lachryma-jobi), *Fu Shen* (Sclerotium Pararadicis Poriae Cocos), *Mu Xiang* (Radix Auklandiae Lappae), *Suan Zao Ren* (Semen Zizyphi Spinosae), *Fang Feng* (Radix Ledebouriellae Divaricatae), *Gan Cao* (Radix Glycyrrhizae), *Du Huo* (Radix Angelicae Pubescentis), *Xing Ren* (Semen Pruni Armeniacae), *Wu Jia Pi* (Cortex Radicis Acanthopanacis), and *Sheng Jiang* (uncooked Rhizoma Zingiberis). *Zhu Ye Tang* (Bamboo Leaf Decoction)

For fetal vexation, drink *Fu Ling* (Sclerotium Poriae Cocos), *Fang Feng* (Radix Ledebouriellae Divaricatae), *Mai Dong* (Tuber Ophiopogonis Japonici), *Huang Qin* (Radix Scutellariae Baicalensis), and *Zhu Ye* (Folium Bambusae). Then one will be quiet and calm asleep or awake.

*Fu Ling Tang* (Poria Decoction)

For fetal swelling, drink *Gan Cao* (Radix Glycyrrhizae), *Fu Ling* (Sclerotium Poriae Cocos), *Chuan Xiong* (Radix Ligustici Wallichii), *Dang Gui* (Radix Angelicae Sinensis), *Bai Shao* (Radix Albus Paeoniae Lactiflorae), *Shu Di* (cooked Radix Rehmanniae), *Huang Qin* (Radix Scutellariae Baicalensis), *Mai Dong* (Tuber Ophiopogonis Japonici), *Zhi Zi* (Fructus Gardeniae Jasminoidis), *Hou Po* (Cortex Magnoliae Officinalis), *Ze Xie* (Rhizoma Alismatis), and *Bai Zhu* (Rhizoma Atractylodis Macrocephalae). Decoct these in water and administer.

*Li Shi Tian Xian Teng San* (Master Li's Aristolochia Stem Powder)

---

[69] *I.e.*, eclampsia gravidarum

For fetal qi[70], use a decoction of *Tian Xian Teng* (Caulis Aristolochiae), *Chen Pi* (Pericarpium Citri Reticulatae), *Xiang Fu* (Rhizoma Cyperi Rotundi), *Zi Su* (Folium Perillae Frutescentis), *Wu Yao* (Radix Linderae Strychnifoliae), *Mu Gua* (Fructus Chaenomelis Lagenariae), *Gan Cao* (Radix Glycyrrhizae), and *Jiang* (Rhizoma Zingiberis).

A woman suffered from malign obstruction[71] in the second month of pregnancy. I used *Er Chen Tang* (Two Aged [Ingredients] Decoction) plus *Dang Gui* (Radix Angelicae Sinensis), *Bai Shao* (Radix Paeoniae Lactiflorae), *Huang Lian* (Rhizoma Coptidis Chinensis), *Bai Zhu* (Rhizoma Atractylodis Macrocephalae), *Zhu Ru* (Caulis Bambusae In Taeniis), and *Wu Mei* (Fructus Pruni Mume) and achieved an instantaneous cure.

(Another) woman suffered from heart pain in the third month of pregnancy. I stir-fried [till red] one *qian* of *Shi Yan* (salt) and stir-fried [till black] fourteen pieces of *Da Zao* (Fructus Zizyphi Jujubae), ground them to powder, and administered these with wine. A cure ensued in no time.

Appendix: *Bao Chan Wu You Tang* (Protect Birth No Worries Decoction)

(This formula) is contained in the *Fu Shi Nu Ke (Master Fu's Gynecology)*, "*Chan Hou Pian Bu Ji* (A Supplement to Postpartum [Diseases]." It is able to quiet (the fetus) before birth and hasten delivery during labor. When the fetal qi is damaged by chance, lumbago and abdominal pain may appear or even red (*i.e.*, blood) is discharged incessantly threatening miscarriage. In such critical occasions, one dose may cure, while another dose can achieve complete recovery. In case of transverse or foot (first) presentation, administration (of this formula) is miraculously effective.

(This formula is composed of) *Dang Gui* (Radix Angelicae Sinensis), *Chuan Xiong* (Radix Ligustici Wallichii), and *Tu Si Zi* (Semen Cuscutae Chinensis), one and a half *qian* each; *Hou Po* (Cortex Magnoliae Officinalis), wine-soaked, and *Jiu Shao* (wine-processed Radix Paeoniae

---

[70] *I. e.*, edematous swelling arising only below the knees in pregnancy.

[71] This refers to vomiting in early pregnancy.

Lactiflorae), two *qian* each; *Zhi Ke* (Fructus Citri Aurantii) and *Qiang Huo* (Radix Et Rhizoma Notopterygii), eight *fen* each; *Bei Mu* (Bulbus Fritillariae), *Jie Sui* (Herba Schizonepetae Tenuifoliae), and *Huang Qi* (Radix Astragali Membranacei), one *qian* each; *Ai Ye* (Folium Artemisiae Argyi) and *Zhi Gan Cao* (mix-fried Radix Glycyrrhizae), five *fen* each; and *Xian Jiang* (fresh Rhizoma Zingiberis) as the conductor.

Notes by Le-tian: Twenty-five years ago, when my wife was in her third month of pregnancy, she slipped one rainy day with some weights on her shoulder and subsequently the fetus was damaged. She suffered from such unbearable abdominal pain that she rolled about on the bed. I administered her the above formula in the prescribed amounts. In a while, she quieted down. Two doses and the condition was cured.

## 74. Postpartum Fever Has Seven Causes

There are seven causes of postpartum fever. There is fever due to excessive loss of blood, fever due to retention of the lochia, fever due to contraction of wind cold, fever due to damage by overeating, fever due to steaming breast milk, fever due to inflated breasts, and fever due to taxation caused by rising up (*i.e.*, going about) too soon after birthing. (Therefore,) it is necessary to inquire about the causes and palpate the pulses. If it is caused by excessive loss of blood, the six pulses must be vacuous. This requires *Yi Qi Yang Ying Tang* (Boost the Qi & Nourish the Constructive Decoction). If it is due to retention of the lochia, there must be abdominal pain. This requires *Hei Shen San* (Black Spirit Powder). If it is due to contraction of wind cold, there must be simultaneous headache. This requires *Wu Ji San* (Five Accumulations Powder). If it is due to damage by overeating, there is constriction of the chest and diaphragm. This requires *Xiao Shi Yin* (Disperse Food Drink). If fever is due to steaming breast milk, the breast milk is not freely flowing. This requires *Tong Ru Tang* (Free the Flow of the Breast Milk Decoction). If fever is due to inflated breasts and there is no one to drink the breast milk, grind five *qian* of *Mai Ya* (Fructus Germinatus Hordei Vulgaris) and take with rice decoction. If it is due to taxation caused by rising up too soon after birthing, there is pain in the lumbus and hips. This requires *Zhu Shen Yin*

(Pig's Kidney Drink). Generally speaking, medicinals used for postpartum (problems) must be warm and, to course and free the flow of the lochia, the ruling (method) is to greatly supplement the qi and blood. Even though there are pathoconditions other (than postpartum ones), these pathoconditions should be treated as the ends (*i.e.*, branches).

*Yi Qi Yang Ying Tang* (Boost the Qi & Nourish the Constructive Decoction)

*Yi Qi Yang Ying Tang* (is composed of) *Ren Shen* (Radix Panacis Ginseng), *Huang Qi* (Radix Astragali Membranacei), *Bai Zhu* (Rhizoma Atractylodis Macrocephalae), *Dang Gui* (Radix Angelicae Sinensis), *Shao Yao* (Radix Paeoniae Lactiflorae), *Chuan Xiong* (Radix Ligustici Wallichii), *Chen Pi* (Pericarpium Citri Reticulatae), and *Shu Di* (cooked Radix Rehmanniae), with *Gan Cao* (Radix Glycyrrhizae) and *Fu Ling* (Sclerotium Poriae Cocos) as assistants.

*Hei Shen San* (Black Spirit Powder)

*Hei Shen San* (is composed of) *Shu Di* (cooked Radix Rehmanniae), stir-fried *Pu Huang* (Pollen Typhae), *Hei Jiang* (blackened Rhizoma Zingiberis), *Chi Shao* (Radix Rubrus Paeoniae Lactiflorae), *Gui Wei* (Extremitas Radicis Angelicae Sinensis), *Rou Gui* (Cortex Cinnamomi Cassiae), *Zhi Gan Cao* (mix-fried Radix Glycyrrhizae), and *Hei Dou* (black Semen Glycineae Hispidae), which is stir-fried till fragrant.

*Wu Ji San* (Five Accumulations Powder)

*Wu Ji* (is composed of) *Chen Pi* (Pericarpium Citri Reticulatae), *Cang Zhu* (Rhizoma Atractylodis), *Bai Zhi* (Radix Angelicae Dahuricae), *Ma Huang* (Herba Ephedrae), *Jie Geng* (Radix Platycodi Grandiflorae), *Fu Ling* (Sclerotium Poriae Cocos), *Gui Zhi* (Ramulus Cinnamomi Cassiae), *Gan Jiang* (dry Rhizoma Zingiberis), *Ban Xia* (Rhizoma Pinelliae Ternatae), *Zhi Ke* (Fructus Citri Aurantii), *Hou Po* (Cortex Magnoliae Officinalis), *Shao Yao* (Radix Paeoniae Lactiflorae), *Dang Gui* (Radix Angelicae Sinensis), and *Chuan Xiong* (Radix Ligustici Wallichii).
*Xiao Shi Yin* (Disperse Food Beverage)

*Xiao Shi Yin* (is composed of) *Shan Zha* (Fructus Crataegi), *Qing Pi* (Pericarpium Citri Reticulatae Viride), *Chen Pi* (Pericarpium Citri Reticulatae), *Shen Qu* (Massa Medica Fermentata), *Mai Ya* (Fructus Germinatus Hordei Vulgaris), *Cang Zhu* (Rhizoma Atractylodis), *Fu Ling* (Sclerotium Poriae Cocos), *Gan Cao* (Radix Glycyrrhizae), *Zhi Shi* (Fructus Immaturus Citri Aurantii), *Hou Po* (Cortex Magnoliae Officinalis), *Mu Xiang* (Radix Auklandiae Lappae), and *Sha Ren* (Fructus Amomi).

*Tong Ru Tang* (Free the Flow of the Breast Milk Decoction)

*Tong Ru Tang* (is composed of) *Tong Cao* (Medulla Tetrapanacis Papyriferi), *Zhu Ti* (pig's foot), *Chuan Xiong* (Radix Ligustici Wallichii), *Gan Cao* (Radix Glycyrrhizae), and *Shan Jia* (Squama Manitis Pentadactylis). Decoct these together and administer and then (milk) will trickle out.

*Zhu Shen Yin* (Pig's Kidney Drink) [a.k.a. *Shi Zi Tang,* Stone Decoction]

*Zhu Shen Yin* (Pig's Kidney Drink) is for delivery taxation. (It includes) *Bai Shao* (Radix Albus Paeoniae Lactiflorae), *Dang Gui* (Radix Angelicae Sinensis), *Jing Mi* (Semen Oryzae Sativae), and *Xiang Chi* (Semen Praeparatus Sojae). *Cong Bai* (Bulbus Allii Fistulosi) is also an ingredient.

# Formula Index

179

# General Index

## A

## B

## C

# OTHER BOOKS ON CHINESE MEDICINE AVAILABLE FROM BLUE POPPY PRESS

1775 Linden Ave, Boulder, CO 80304
For ordering 1-800-487-9296 PH. 303\447-8372 FAX 303\447-0740

**A NEW AMERICAN ACUPUNCTURE** by Mark Seem, ISBN 0-936185-44-9

**ACUPUNCTURE AND MOXIBUSTION FORMULAS & TREATMENTS** by Cheng Dan-an, trans. by Wu Ming, ISBN 0-936185-68-6,

**ACUTE ABDOMINAL SYNDROMES: Their Diagnosis & Treatment by Combined Chinese-Western Medicine** by Alon Marcus, ISBN 0-936185-31-7

**AGING & BLOOD STASIS: A New Approach to TCM Geriatrics** by Yan De-xin, ISBN 0-936185-63-5

**AIDS & ITS TREATMENT ACCORDING TO TRADITIONAL CHINESE MEDICINE** by Huang Bing-shan, trans. by Fu-Di & Bob Flaws, ISBN 0-936185-28-7

**ARISAL OF THE CLEAR: A Simple Guide to Healthy Eating According to Traditional Chinese Medicine,** Bob Flaws, ISBN #-936185-27-9

**THE BOOK OF JOOK: Chinese Medicinal Porridges, An Alternative to the Typical Western Breakfast** by Bob Flaws, ISBN0-936185-60-0

**CHINESE MEDICAL PALMISTRY: Your Health in Your Hand** by Zong Xiao-fan & Gary Liscum, ISBN 0-936185-64-3

**CHINESE MEDICINAL TEAS: Simple, Proven, Folk Formulas for Common Diseases & Promoting Health** by Zong Xiao-fan & Gary Liscum, ISBN 0-936185-76-7

**CHINESE MEDICINAL WINES & ELIXIRS** by B. Flaws, ISBN 0-936185-58-9

**CHINESE PEDIATRIC MASSAGE THERAPY: A Parent's & Practitioner's Guide to the Prevention & Treatment of Childhood Illness** by Fan Ya-li, ISBN 0-936185-54-6

**CHINESE SELF-MASSAGE THERAPY: The Easy Way to Health** by Fan Ya-li ISBN 0-936185-74-0

**CLASSICAL MOXIBUSTION SKILLS in Clinical Practice** by Sung Baek, ISBN 0-936185-16-3

**A COMPENDIUM OF TCM PATTERNS & TREATMENTS** by Bob Flaws & Daniel Finney, ISBN 0-936185-70-8

**THE DAO OF INCREASING LONGEVITY AND CONSERVING ONE'S LIFE** by Anna Lin & Bob Flaws, ISBN 0-936185-24-4

**THE DIVINELY RESPONDING CLASSIC: A Translation of the Shen Ying Jing from Zhen Jiu Da Cheng,** trans. by Yang Shou-zhong & Liu Feng-ting ISBN 0-936185-55-4

**ENDOMETRIOSIS, INFERTILITY AND TRADITIONAL CHINESE MEDICINE: A Laywoman's Guide** by Bob Flaws ISBN 0-936185-14-7